Barriers to Breast Cancer Prevention and Screening among African American Women

By

Abosede Francisca Obikunle

Published by: JB Books

ISBN: 979-8-9870384-1-3

Abstract

Breast cancer is a serious illness that often has fatal consequences. Adherence to the recommendations for breast cancer surveillance is poorly practiced among African American women. The purpose of this phenomenological study was to seek individual professed barriers to breast cancer screening among African American women to better understand why breast cancer continues to be one of the principal basis of mortality among African American women. The theoretical framework for this study was the behavioral model of health services use. Purposeful selection was used to invite 14 African American women to participate in the in-depth interview process. Interview data were transcribed and then coded for recurring themes and meaning. The findings of this study demonstrate that these women's perceived barriers to breast cancer screening were lack of information, a belief that genetics dictates who gets breast cancer, embarrassment, a norm of people not going for health checkups, the procedure of breast cancer screening, and fear. Participants noted that the improved method of mammography may promote utilization within the population. Breast cancer disparities among African American women may decline if healthcare providers promote awareness of the availability and accessibility of breast cancer prevention resources and if African American women understand the barriers to breast cancer prevention and change their own screening practices.

Dedication

I would like to dedicate this book to all the women of the world that will elude breast cancer through their adherence to the recommendations for breast cancer prevention and the utilization of the available resources. I also dedicate this project to all the survivors of breast cancer, the women currently suffering from breast cancer and to the memory of those who died from breast cancer.

Acknowledgments

I would like to acknowledge my committee Chair, Dr. Diane Cortner, and my committee member, Dr. Janice Williams, for their prompt scholarly advice and support.

My special thanks go to God for His mercy that endures forever. Thanks to my husband Femi and our children Tomi, Tolu, Temi and Tani for their support and understanding. I would also like to acknowledge my friends, Kayode, Yinka, Frank, Muyiwa, Odun, Charles, Tina, Tiya and Alaba (RIP) who offered me their feedback throughout this project. I would also like to acknowledge the cooperation of my study participants in the completion of this project and thanks to everyone who directly or indirectly contributed to the success of the study which culminated in this book.

Table of Contents

List of Tables

List of Figures

Chapter 1:

Introduction to the Study

Introduction

Breast cancer is a predominant non-skin cancer in females and has emerged as one of the leading causes of mortality among women in the United States (American Cancer Society [ACS], 2011; Jemal et al., 2005). Although immense progress has been made in screening procedures and mammography practices for the general population, lesser screening rates are seen in various female subgroups (ACS, 2011; U.S. Department of Health and Human Services, Centers for Disease Control and Prevention [CDC], 2013). Women from ethnic minority communities have a tendency to present as diagnosed with tumors at a later phase of cancer. This disparity has been attributed to the fact that minority women lack adequate knowledge about early screening detection services for breast cancer (CDC, 2013).

Lower screening participation amongst African American women are known to be the result of barriers at the personal and system level that are inversely linked with the rate of breast cancer screening (Deavenport, Modeste, Marshak, & Neish, 2011). Personal barriers include psychological implications that hinder the choice to obtain mammography, while system barriers include difficulties in accessing health care facilities and the cost and affordability of breast screening by mammogram (Ahmed, Fort, Fair, Semenya, & Haber, 2009; Oh, Zhou, Kreps & Rvu, 2012; van den Biggelaar, Kessels, van Engelshoven, & Flobbe, 2009).

Despite efforts to reduce prevailing disparities, limited information is available regarding differences in screening practices between various ethnic groups.

African American women are known to have inexplicably higher incidence of breast cancer mortality than European American women, in spite of having a lower occurrence rate. Although screening rates are increasing for African American women, breast cancer is often diagnosed at late stages in this population, which limits the treatment options (ACS, 2013a). The goal of the present study is to understand prevailing barriers to breast cancer screening among African American women. Few studies have targeted African American women for breast cancer surveillance in an effort to reduce this health disparity.

Furthermore, no studies have explored how personal barriers, stereotypes, socioeconomic status, culture, attitudes, and beliefs may influence the behavior of African American women in regard to preventive approaches to breast cancer. Without exploring the factors affecting breast cancer routine testing among African American women, breast cancer will continue to be a great contributory factor to mortality in this population. The findings of this study may contribute to interventions that increase access to screening programs that have the ability to detect tumors at early stages and hence reduce health disparities within the population. Phenomenological inquiry was used to explore the influence of personal barriers, stereotypes, socioeconomic status, culture, attitudes, and beliefs on the outlook of African American women in regard to breast cancer screening.

A phenomenological approach will be used for this study to better understand the individual professed barriers to breast cancer screening among African American women and why breast cancer continues to be one of the principal bases of mortality in African American women. In the theoretical framework, the behavioral model of health services use will be described and will be a guide for this study.

Chapter 1 provides the barriers to breast cancer prevention among African American women, the research problem statement, purpose of the study, and the research questions. It also details the significance of the study and its implications for social change and the description of operational definitions, delimitations, assumptions, and limitations.

Background

Cancer is a deadly disease that affects a large number of people per year in the United States (Lin & Plevritis, 2012). The majority of cancer cells ultimately become a lump, which is described as a tumor in an anatomical position with respect to the original location. Breast cancer starts in breast tissues comprised of lobules. A lump in the breast may be detected during routine screening prior to the development of symptoms, or after the development of symptoms, when a woman detects a lump. In most cases, masses observed on a mammogram are benign or noncancerous i.e., not life threatening (ACS, 2013a). However, for cancer cases that are suspected on the basis of breast imaging or clinical breast examination (CBE), microscopic examination of the mammary glands is essential for an ultimate conclusion and to understand the degree of invasion into healthy tissue (ACS, 2013a). Early detection of this disease through screening and tests could be lifesaving (Kadivar et al., 2012).

Breast cancer is the most prevailing of all the malignancies across the world and is distinguished by early inception and late diagnosis (ACS, 2013a). Accordingly, promoting awareness among women of the importance of screening is essential for decreasing the rate of mortality (Kadivar et al., 2012).

Various risk factors are associated with breast cancer. For example, early onset of menarche, delivery of one's first baby after the age of 30, and never having children are higher contributory factors to emergent breast cancer (ACS, 2009). Other risk factors for women include the inheritance of a single imperfect copy of any of the cancer suppressor genes, *BRCA1* and *BRCA2*. Conversely, the production of cancerous cells is a multifaceted chain that takes place in several separate stages that typically involve a great number of genetic changes. In addition, there are other non-genetic influences on gene expression that are accountable for carcinogenesis which include hormone levels, and exposure to cancer-causing substances or agent and tumor support agents. Non-genetic factors are not necessarily cancer- producing agents; however, they enhance the chances of hereditary gene alterations that result in malignant cells (Katzung, Masters, & Trevor, 2009). The *BRCA-1*, *BRCA-2*, *p53*, *ATM* (ataxia telangienctasia mutated), and *HER-2/neu* oncogenes are the major contributing genes for the development of breast cancer. The degree of amplification is an important factor in determining survival time of the patient and the chances of cancer relapse; early detection prevents major loss (Cancer Research UK, 2013).

Obesity has been associated with greater risk of breast cancer among postmenopausal African American women (Sarkissyan, Wu, & Vadgama, 2011). Obesity rates are higher among African American women in comparison to European American women–53% versus 37%, respectively (U.S Department of Health and Human Services [DHS], National Center for Health Statistics [NCHS], 2009). Additionally, lesser number of morbidly overweight women tend to participate in, and report, current mammography screening (NCHS, 2009). Obesity is likely to support faster and wider spread of cancer due to damaged cellular immunity (Sarkissyan et al., 2011). Hyperinsulinemia, which is prevalent in obese women, increases the level of leptin and insulin-like growth factor, which may promote mammary carcinogenesis. This is through a synergistic effect with estrogen that promotes angiogenesis in the epithelial cells of mammary glands (Cohen et al., 2008).

According to the National Health Interview Survey (Swan et al., 2010), 67% of women in middle age reported to have participated in mammogram screening within the last 2 years. Breen, Gentlemen, and Schiller (2011) reported that mammography prevalence increased from 29% in 1987 to 70% in 2000. A slight decline of 3.4% was observed between 2000 and 2005, but this has gradually stabilized. Breen et al (2011) also reported that women who (a) have low levels of education—for example, less than a high school education, (b) do not have insurance coverage, or (c) have recently immigrated to the United States, are known to have not participated in mammogram screening in the last 2 years.

Women of low socioeconomic status are less than likely to have had a mammogram in the last 2 years as compared to affluent women, and denial of mammography screening is observed more in poor women. Screening should be encouraged for this disadvantaged group of women, as they are known to have the lowest rates of mammographic screening (ACS, 2013a).

From 1975 to 1990, breast cancer rates increased at the rate of 0.4% per year, while mortality rates declined by 34% from 1990 to 2010 (Howlader et al., 2013). The reduction in mortality occurred at a faster rate in women under 50 compared to women aged 50 and above (3.1% versus 1.9% per year, respectively). From 2001 to 2010, the incidence rate for African American women's mortality declined slower than that for non-Hispanic European American women (1.6% versus 1.8%, respectively) (Howlader et al., 2013) and other ethnic communities

(ACS, 2013a). The significant drop in breast cancer mortality rates for all groups is due to advancements in breast cancer treatment and timely discovery of cancer cells. However, from the 1980s, disparities in breast cancer mortality rates have been observed. In 2010, breast cancer mortality among African American women aged 45 to 64 years was 60% greater than for European American women (56.8 vs. 35.6 deaths per 100,000, respectively) (Black Women's Health Imperative, n.d.). This gap reflects the earlier uptake of diagnostic steps and higher prevalence of mammography among European American women. In addition, differences have been observed in regard to access to new advances in treatment, such as tamoxifen.

Tamoxifen is used for the treatment of hormone-receptor-positive breast cancers, which are less prevalent among African American women. Few studies have addressed targeting African American women for breast cancer surveillance in efforts to reduce these health disparities (Smith et al., 2010). Although the prevalence of breast cancer is lesser in African American women in comparison to European American women, mortality rates are higher (van Ravesteyn et al., 2011).

In the analysis of a 5-year continued existence rate for European American women compared to African American women, the result showed a rate of 90% to 77% respectively (Black Women's Health Imperative, n.d.). Various reasons for these disparities exist. For example, breast cancer is likely to appear at an earlier age in African American women and in a more advanced form. Reports reveal that African American women are two times more likely to develop the more aggressive form of breast cancer, called triple negative breast cancer (TNBC) (Thompson et al., 2009). TNBC spreads and grows more rapidly than any other form of breast cancer, and the condition has less efficacious treatment options. In addition, African American breast cancer survivors show lower compliance rates with post treatment surveillance compared to European American women survivors (Thompson et al., 2009). African American women have thicker and more complex breast tissue, a very high predictor of breast cancer risk, and this limits the sensitivity of breast screening through mammograms (Black Women's Health Imperative, n.d.). Small tumors may remain undetected, and symptoms of breast cancer are absent in the early stages.

However, regular screening remains important for this group because breast cancer is treatable when detected early (Black Women's Health Imperative, n.d.). The present study was carried out to understand the barriers to breast cancer screening experienced by African American women.

Several studies have identified barriers to breast cancer screening and prevention among African American women. The most commonly identified barriers include lack of education (Gullatte et al., 2010; Breen et al., 2011), lack of awareness (Kadivar et al., 2012), and inappropriate health insurance due to poverty (Hoffman et al., 2011). In addition, attending religious services and deriving comfort through prayers or reading Biblical scriptures is becoming more prevalent among African American breast cancer survivors, which contributes to poor adherence to post treatment regimens (Lynn, Yoo, & Levine, 2013). However, few of these studies have explored the problems in the perspective of the behavioral model of health services use (BMHSU) to understand the predisposing, enabling, and need-related factors of African American women. The present study uses the BMHSU framework to explore personal barriers to breast cancer screening among African American women. The study aims to advance interventions for enhancing the access of African American women to screening programs such as mammography in order to detect tumors at earlier stages and reduce mortality associated with breast cancer.

Problem Statement

No studies have explored how personal barriers, stereotypes, socioeconomic status, culture, attitudes, and beliefs may influence the behavior of African American women in regard to preventive approaches to breast cancer. Without the research evidence to explain this phenomenon, targeted interventions may be ineffective (Summers et al., 2010).

Breast cancer is a common cancer in women across the world (ACS, 2011; Heiney, 2014). Early detection enhances patient survival rates (Cancer Research UK, 2010; Summers, Saltzstein, Blair, Tsukamoto, & Sadler, 2010). However, screening rates among African American women are low. Delays in accessing health care services result in breast cancers being detected at later stages. The reasons for such delays involve psychological and social factors (Heisey et al., 2011). Among African American women, personal barriers such as attitudes, beliefs, sociocultural background, and personality of the individual directly influence interpretation of symptoms, the decision to seek health care and social interactions to access support from allied health services (Viswanathan et al., 2009). Research that focuses on reducing breast cancer mortality amongst African American women should also include sociocultural investigations of barriers to screening and prevention (Summers et al., 2010). Breast cancer is one of the leading causes of mortality in African American women (ACS, 2011; Summers et al., 2010). Breast cancer prevention among African American women can be enhanced through improved awareness, surveillance, and follow-up health care for survivors (Thompson et al., 2009).

No studies have focused on the perspectives of African American women regarding personal barriers, attitudes, and beliefs in regard to breast cancer and screening. Understanding barriers to breast cancer screening among African American women will help healthcare providers improve healthcare services for this population and address the issue of healthcare disparities among women.

Purpose of the Study

Barriers to breast cancer screening may be categorized as structural, clinical, or personal. Structural barriers include low socioeconomic status and inadequate accessibility to a high standard of care (Peek, Sayad, & Markwardt, 2008) or preventive health care services (Conway-Phillips & Million-Underwood, 2009). Clinical barriers arise once women do not get screened, either due to negative interactions with caregivers (Peek et al., 2008) or having received inadequate information from care providers regarding breast cancer screening (Conway-Phillips & Million Underwood, 2009). Personal barriers—such as a lack of knowledge about breast cancer or lack of trust in the healthcare system—are directly proportional to limited breast cancer awareness (Frisby, 2012; Gullatte et al., 2010).

According to Amanda Phipps, a postdoctoral fellow at the Fred Hutchinson Cancer Research Center, "Breast cancer is not just one disease. It is a complex combination of many diseases" (American Association of Cancer Research, 2011, para. 3). Breast cancer is a multifaceted condition consisting of divergent biological subtypes with dissimilar natural histories. Consequently, breast cancer presents as a wide-ranging spectrum of pathological, clinical, and molecular features with diverse therapeutic and prognostic propositions (Onitilo, Engel, Greenlee, & Mukesh, 2009). Breast cancer characteristically does not produce any symptoms at the initial stages, that is, when the tumor is minute and could be cured easily. Thus, screening is critical for early detection and successful treatment.

In the United States, 1 in every 8 women is diagnosed with breast cancer (ACS, 2013a). In the 1970s, this ratio was 1 in 11. The increase in incidence has been attributed to changes in lifestyle, longer life expectancy, and changes in reproductive patterns, use of menopausal hormones, increased obesity, and increased detection through screening (ACS, 2013a). African American women under 40 are known to have much higher incidence rate of breast cancer than European American women and have higher risk of mortality rate (ACS, 2013a).

Russell, Monahan, Wagle, and Champion (2006) reported that African American women with (a) relatively low-income, (b) awareness of breast cancer vulnerability, (c) the advantages of screening, and (d) the barriers to screening were stage-specific. Pre-contemplators (not planning to have a mammogram) displayed poor knowledge, the lowest apparent advantages, and maximum barrier scores, while contemplators (planning to have a mammogram) were apprehensive about finding a lump.

Among African American women, the decision to seek preventative screening for breast cancer is related to perceived risk, cultural beliefs, and other barriers. Recognized beliefs include fear of cancer detection, fear of doctors, and fear of treatment (Shigematsu et al., 2010). In addition, a fatalistic view persists among African American women about the predictability of demise once cancer is identified. Certain folk beliefs also prevail, such as the belief that breast cancer surgery causes the cancer to spread or that a lump is the result of a sore or bruise. Folk remedial measures (Sheppard et al., 2013), nontraditional cancer treatments (Yoo, Kreuter, Lai, & Fu, 2013), collectivism (Taylor et al., 2012; Tejeda et al., 2013), and social networks (McQueen, Kreuter, Kalesan, & Alcaraz, 2011; Swinney & Dobal, 2011; Zollinger et al., 2010) also play a role in the decision to seek preventative screening for breast cancer.

The purpose of this research was to identify barriers to preventative screening for breast cancer among African American women. This study employed a qualitative phenomenological approach to explore the influence of personal barriers, stereotypes, socioeconomic status, culture, attitudes, and beliefs on the behavior of African American women in regard to breast cancer screening. The findings of this study may contribute to interventions that increase access to screening programs that can detect tumors at early stages and hence reduce health disparities within the population.

Research Questions

The following research question contains one central question and two sub-questions.

RQ: What are the perceived barriers for breast cancer screening among African American Women?

Sub-RQ1: How can awareness of breast cancer screening and prevention be promoted among African American women?

Sub-RQ2: How does stereotype and culture influence African American women's beliefs and behavior in regard to breast cancer screening and prevention?

Theoretical Framework

The theoretical framework for this study was the behavioral model of health services use (BMHSU) (Andersen, 1995). It was originally developed in the late 1960s to aid in understanding how and why families use health services. Andersen's behavioral model of utilization is among the most commonly used frameworks for evaluating issues linked with patients' use of wellness services. Health care utilization is the point at which the patient's needs are compared to the expertise of the healthcare providers and the available resources in the health systems. Health care utilization is strongly based on the composition of the health care system, and patient's needs and is supply-induced. According to the model, the decision of an individual to use health care services is determined, at least in part, by predisposing, enabling, and need-related factors (Andersen, 1995; Manski et al., 2013).

Predisposing Factors

Factors that predispose an individual to the use of medical services include (a) biological imperatives, for example, a person's age and sex, (b) social factors such as occupation, education, family status, ethnicity, and (c) mental factors and beliefs which include a person's values, attitudes, and their knowledge about health services (Babitsch, Gohl, & von Lengerke, 2012, p. 7). Other factors include cultural values, political views, the social composition and demographics of the community, and the organizational values upheld by the society (Babitsch et al., 2012).

Enabling Factors

The use of services depends on organizational as well as fiscal factors. These two factors create an enabling environment for the use of service. A person's disposable income and wealth status determine their ability to meet their health costs (Summers et al., 2010). At the same time, the ability of an individual to meet the price of healthcare is determined by the cost-sharing agreement between an individual and their insurance companies (Babitsch et al., 2012). Organizational factors include travel time to the health facility, means of transportation, and the waiting time at the hospital before one gets treated (Andersen, 1995). Hence, these factors determine whether an individual has access to a constant source of care and the characteristics of that source. Contextually, financing for health services is determined by the factors that are available within the reach of the community These factors include, but are not limited to, per capita income, prices for goods and services, wealth status, individual health insurance coverage, methods used by insurance, providers in compensation, and health care expenditures (Babitsch et al., 2012). At this level, the term *organization* refers to the structures, quantity, distribution, locations, and types of health services facilities. It also refers to the provider mix, quality management oversight, hospital personnel, physician and hospital density, office hours for consultations, and outreach and educational programs.

Need factors

At the individual level, Andersen tries to differentiate between the evaluated and the perceived need for health services (Andersen, 1995). The evaluated need refers to how people view and determine their own general health, sickness symptoms, and their ordinary functional states. The evaluated need is the attending physician's professional assessment, the objective, and subjective measurements of patients' health status, and need for medical care. At the contextual level, need factors help in differentiating between population health and environmental factors. Environmental characteristics such as crime-related, traffic, and occupational injuries resulting in death reflect the health-related conditions of the environment. Population health indices measure the community health status though factors such as the rate of disability, morbidity, and mortality (Babitsch et al., 2012). However, even to this day, no studies have been conducted to examine the views of African American women on the influence of beliefs, culture, stereotypes and personal barriers, attitudes, and socioeconomic status on breast cancer screening. This study delves into these issues using a phenomenological method to identify hindrances to breast cancer screening among African American women.

Nature of the Study

This study used a qualitative approach to explore the perspectives of African American women regarding the influence of personal barriers, stereotypes, socioeconomic status, culture, attitudes, and beliefs about breast cancer screening. Fourteen African American women made up the sample in an effort to better understand their attitudes and behaviors in regard to breast cancer screening. The theoretical framework for this study was the BMHSU (Andersen, 1995). The model was originally developed in the late 1960s to increase understanding of why families use health services (Andersen, 1995, p-1). The BMHSU asserted that the use of health care services by a person is partly determined by predisposing, enabling, and need factors (Manski et al., 2013).

Definitions

African American: People having origin in any of the Black racial groups of the United States, Africa or other parts of the world.

Breast Cancer: Cancer that forms in lobules (glands that make milk), and the

ducts (tubes that carry milk to the nipple). It occurs usually in women with rare occurrence in men (NCI, 2013)

Breast Self-Examination (BSE): A self-examination of a woman's breasts to check for lumps and other changes (ACS, 2013a).

Cancer: Cancer is a deadly disease that affects over one million people per year in the United States when untreated. Ultimately, it can cause death (Lin & Plevritis, 2012).

Clinical Breast Examination (CBE): A physical examination of the breast performed by a healthcare provider to check for lumps and other changes (ACS, 2013a).

Ducts: Breast tubules that carry milk to the nipples (NCI, 2013).

Early Detection: Timely discovery of cancer cells which could promote increased survival rate. Evidence implies that early detection reduces the likelihood of higher mortality from cancer (Kadivar et al., 2012).

Ethnic Group (Ethnicity): A representative of a number of people who identify with each other through a familiar inheritance, including a general language and traditions (Komenaka et al., 2010).

Health Behavior: Individual's characteristic such as values, attitude, objective, values, and awareness, emotional states and traits that contribute to health choices (Ahmadian, & Samah, 2013).

Health Disparities: Variation in the occurrence, frequency, mortality, and other unfavorable health issues that are present within a particular population (Hoffman et al., 2011; Komenaka et al., 2010).

Interpretative phenomenology approach (IPA): One of the six essential types of phenomenology approach. A phenomenology provides a deep understanding of a phenomenon as experienced by several individuals" (Creswell, 2007, p. 62)

Mammography: Picture of the breast through an X-ray or film typically for detection of tumors (van Ravesteyn et al., 2011).

Minority Groups: Division of group of the people that consist of less than 50% of the population (Hoffman et al., 2011).

Assumptions

The assumptions associated with this study included the following: (a) study procedures were adequate to achieve accurate data from the sample population, (b) participants would be honest and accurate (c) the sample was assumed to be representative of African American women.

Scope

In this study the sample was comprised of 14 African American women living in an urban East Coast region. Interviews were used to gather information in order to understand African American women's professed personal barriers, stereotype, socio-economic status, culture, attitudes, beliefs, and how these factors influenced breast cancer screening.

Delimitations

This study centered on the fact that only African American women from a community in a local church in an urban East Coast region were purposefully sampled and interviewed.

Limitations

Purposeful sampling was the method of choice for this study. However, using this method limited the extent of generalizability since the sample of African American women from a local religious center may not necessarily represent the general population of African American women. The data are personal and thus may bear little relationship to the views of others. In addition, confidence about individual reports as the principal means of data collection was another limitation. I can only presume that participants responded to interview questions accurately and truthfully. Despite the disadvantages of self-report, it has an advantage: Self-report gave the researcher the respondents' own view directly. In addition, advantages such as convenience, cost-effectiveness, and participants answering the exact same questions makes self-report a reliable source of data collection.

Significance

The current study aims to help identify the obstacles to preventative breast cancer screening for African American women. The identification of these barriers may help improve their positive screening behaviors. Because early screening means better outcomes, especially for these women who tend to develop the more aggressive types of cancer, lives may thereby be saved. Positive social change may result when African American women understand the barriers to breast cancer prevention and seek to change their own breast cancer screening practices. Healthcare providers should also focus on promoting awareness on the availability and accessibility of breast cancer prevention resources among African American women hence reducing breast cancer disparities.

Summary

The relative frequency of deaths by breast cancer among African American women is significant. However, African American women often get breast cancer diagnosis at an advanced phase, which reduces survival outcomes. In addition, the cancer most often detected in this group of women is TNBC, an aggressive cancer that is difficult to treat. The situation for African American women is further compromised by low screening rates due to various limitations among this population. Awareness of the barriers that prevent African American women from adopting screening behaviors may contribute to improved screening rates for breast cancer, earlier detection, and better survival outcomes for African American women.

Chapter 2 includes a review of literature from peer-reviewed journals published within the last 5 years. The review includes an overview of studies focused on the differential barriers to health and health care facilities that prevent African American women from obtaining timely screening and diagnoses for breast cancer. This chapter explores the methods and procedures for studying African American women's professed personal barriers, stereotype, socioeconomic status, culture, attitudes, beliefs, and how these factors may influence breast cancer screening. Chapter 3 of this study provides a justification for the selected research design, methodology, instrumentation, participants, and methods for data analysis, as well as a discussion of measures of validity and reliability. Chapter 4 covers the results of pilot study, setting, demographics of participants, the data analysis and results. Finally, Chapter 5 covers a discussion based on the results as well as relative conclusions and recommendations.

Chapter 2:
Literature Review

Introduction

Breast cancer occurs in the tissues of the breast. The major category of breast cancer is ductal carcinoma (ACS, 2013a; ACS, 2015). This cancer originates in the inside layer of the milk ducts, which are responsible for carrying milk from the lobules of the breast (the milk glands) to the nipples. Another form of breast cancer is lobular carcinoma, which commences in the lobules. Invasive breast cancer is a kind of breast cancer that spreads from its site of origin to adjoining, noncancerous tissues (Mousavi, Försti, Sundquist, & Hemminki, 2013). Breast cancer occurs predominantly in females (National Institutes of Health, National Cancer Institute [NCI], 2013).

Breast cancer is far-reaching in women across the world. The condition is all the more devastating for African American women as they face various screening barriers. Screening is significant for prompt breast cancer diagnosis, which improves survival outcomes over diagnosis at an advanced stage of the disease. Thus, increasing breast cancer screening opportunities for African American women is critical for improving survival rates among this population (NCI, 2013). This chapter presents a review of the relevant literature in order to provide a contextual background for the present study, a study that aims to identify the barriers prevalent among African American women that prevent them from getting breast cancer screening.

In this chapter, the literature search strategies that were used, the major themes found in the literature and a justification for the selected research methodology are described.

Search Strategy

The present study focuses on the differential barriers to health and health care facilities that prevent African American women from obtaining timely screening and diagnoses for breast cancer. PubMed and MEDLINE databases were searched using the following terms and phrases in various combinations: *barriers to breast cancer screening, African American women, stage at diagnosis, mammography, spirituality, cultural barriers, poverty, social injustice, disparity, underserved, survival and mortality due to breast cancer,* and *socioeconomic status.* Search results were limited to articles published between 2009 and 2014. Approximately 100 articles were identified as relevant to breast cancer screening barriers among African American women, with 84 of them forming part of the reference list.

Breast Cancer

Malignant tumors, if not controlled, can lead to death. Accordingly, timely care and management of cancer is critical to survival (ACS, 2013a; NCI, 2013). Numerous external and internal factors are responsible for the promotion and proliferation of cancer cells. External factors such as tobacco consumption, infectious organisms, exposure to chemicals and radiation, and poor nutrition may induce the uncontrolled propagation of cancerous cells. On the other hand, various internal features that lead to the development of cancer include genetic mutation, metabolic and hormonal alterations, and immune status (ACS, 2013a). These factors may function alone or in conjunction with a combination of other factors to initiate the proliferation of cancer.

The incubation period, which is the time between exposure to external factors and detection of cancer, may last as long as 10 years (ACS, 2013a). Surgery, chemotherapy, radiation therapy, hormone therapy, targeted therapy, and biologic therapy are the most common cancer treatments (ACS, 2013b).

According to the National Cancer Institute (NCI, 2008), disparities in cancer health can be defined as:

Adverse differences in cancer incidence (new cases), cancer prevalence (all existing cases), cancer death (mortality), cancer survivorship, and burden of cancer or related health conditions that exist among specific population groups in the United States (p. 1)

These population groups can be categorized on the basis of age, ethnicity, disability, and gender, level of education, geographic location, race, or income. For example, individuals with low incomes are often deprived of health benefits and insurance and are medically underserved. Ethnicity and racial background also contribute to disparities, including a greater burden of cancer compared to the general population (NCI, 2008).

Among racial and cultural groups in the United States, African Americans have the highest mortality rates and shortest survival periods for most cancers. In 2009, the percentage of mortalities due to cancer among African American was 7% compared to 4% for European American (ACS, 2013b). This situation is largely due to social and economic disparities. Inequalities in work, income, wealth, education, living standards, and housing serve as barriers to the prevention of cancer and its early detection and treatment (ACS, 2013b).

Most cancer cells eventually become a lump, or a mass of cells called a tumor. Breast cancer originates in the breast tissue, which is comprised of the glands, or lobules, that produce milk, the ducts that joins the lobules to the nipple, and connective, fatty, and lymphatic tissues (ACS, 2013a). Breast cancer can be detected during screening examinations well before the development of symptoms.

A mammogram detects masses or lumps in the breast and categorizes them as cancerous or noncancerous (Khaliq, Visvanathan, Landis, & Wright, 2013). Early detection is beneficial for the prevention of mortality due to breast cancer. When breast cancer is suspected on the basis of a mammogram report, CBE, or breast imaging, samples of breast tissue are examined using microscopic analysis in order to establish a definitive diagnosis, verify the extent of the spread of cancerous cells, and characterize the pattern of the disease (ACS, 2013a; Khaliq et al., 2013) Awareness of the importance of BSE and CBE during routine visits to wellness facilities plays a vital role in breast cancer screening (ACS, 2013a).

Women with no family history of breast cancer are less likely to develop breast cancer compared to women having affected first-degree relatives which includes one's parent, sibling, or child (Zhang et al., 2012). This risk is increased when the first-degree relative is younger than 50 years of age. The chances increase further with a greater number of first-degree relatives that have been diagnosed with breast cancer (Zhang et al., 2012). Research shows that screening mammography for women between 39 and 69 years of age reduces breast cancer mortality (Nelson et al., 2009). Mammography and CBE play a vital role in breast cancer detection for susceptible populations of women. For women with a familial risk of breast cancer, regular mammograms, CBE, or BSE are recommended for those under 50 (Zhang et al., 2012).

In some cases, risk of breast cancer may not be related to family history. 64% of women aged 40 to 49 who were diagnosed with invasive breast cancer denied family history of breast cancer compared to 63% who had a history of breast cancer in their family (BreastCancer.org, 2011). These findings imply that family history may not be a contributory factor for breast cancer among younger women. Nevertheless, the general consensus is that woman between the ages of 40 and 50 years should have regular breast exams (BreastCancer.org, 2011).

Breast cancer is considered the most prevalent non-skin cancer in females and has emerged as the second leading cause of mortality among women in the United States (ACS, 2011; Jemal et al., 2010). Although immense progress has been made in screening procedures and mammography practices for the general population, lesser screening rates are seen in various female subgroups (ACS, 2011; CDC, 2013). Breast cancer is predominantly burdensome for African American women (ACS, 2011). Statistics from 2007 to 2009 revealed that the lifetime probability of developing invasive breast cancer was lower for African American women (10.87%, or 1 in 9) compared to 12.73% (1 in 8) for European American women (ACS, 2011). On the other hand, 3.25% (1 in 31) of African American women die of breast cancer compared to 2.73% (1 in 37) of European American women. Thus, while European American women develop cancer at higher rates than African American women, the mortality rate is higher in the latter group.

Disparities in incidence versus mortality rates suggest the existence of preventive factors that diminish breast cancer mortality rates for European American, but not African American, women (Sail, Franzini, Lairson, & Du, 2012).

African American women are predisposed to be diagnosed with more advanced stages of breast cancer compared to European American women, which is a leading cause of breast cancer mortality (Sail et al.; 2012). Batina et al. (2013) looked at racial differences in tumor natural history to determine whether that played a role in survival rates.

The authors reported that mean tumor growth rates were 63.3% faster for African Americans compared to European Americans. Moreover, the tumors were found to be more aggressive, metastasizing at a rate that was 2.2 times higher in African Americans compared to European Americans. Based on these findings, Batina et al. (2013) emphasized the importance of increased access to mammography for the prevention and early detection of breast cancer to eliminate prevailing breast cancer disparities. Suggestions that minority women are not well informed or possess inadequate knowledge about the early screening of detection services for breast cancer have been put forward to explain these health disparities (CDC, 2013). The ACS has guidelines, based on a woman's age, for the early diagnosis of breast cancer that includes mammography, CBE, and magnetic resonance imaging (MRI) (ACS, 2013a).

Breast Cancer Screening

The three primary means of breast cancer screening are mammography, CBE, and BSE (CDC, 2013). The American Cancer Society advocates for yearly mammograms for women aged 40 years and above and breast examinations every 3 years for women between the ages of 20 and 30 years. Generating awareness in women about the benefits of breast screening is particularly important; any changes related to health and breast feel must be reported (ACS, 2013a). Lower screening rates among

African American women have been attributed to barriers at the personal and system level that are inversely associated with the rate of breast cancer screening (Deavenport et al., 2011). Personal barriers include psychological implications that hinder the choice to obtain mammography, while system barriers include difficulties in accessing health care facilities and the cost and affordability of breast screening by mammogram (Ahmed et al., 2009).

Preventive habits, such as mammography, BSE, and CBE, should be promoted as part of every woman's lifestyle. The ACS (2013a) formulated breast cancer screening guidelines for women belonging to different age groups on the basis that early intervention and diagnosis enhance survival rates and, therefore, must be promoted. Essentially, African American women must know the risk factors associated with breast cancer and the diagnosis procedure, including appropriate screening tools for detection.

Hughes (2013) noted that the majority of women lack sufficient knowledge about the threat of breast cancer. European American women have the tendency to hold in too great esteem their risk of breast cancer, which becomes a cause of anxiety, while African American women tend to underrate their risk and, therefore, underutilize available screening resources. Overall, 90.6% women in general do not have adequate knowledge of their own breast cancer risk. In her article, Hughes quoted Dr. Jonathan Herman as saying, "Our education messaging is far off and we should change the way breast cancer awareness is presented" (para. 3).

Hughes (2013) reported on an unpublished survey of African Americans involving questions related to ethnicity, religious, education, affiliation, income, marital status, health insurance, and personal risk issues such as age during first menstrual cycle, age of first delivery (of a child), family and individual history of breast cancer.

The projected risk of breast cancer at age 90 years was determined and compared to subjects' own estimates of their risk. Results from the sample of 781 African Americans showed that only 8.7% of respondents accurately assessed their risk. In contrast, 57.6% of the participants underrated their risk and 33.7% overrated their risk (Hughes, 2013). Furthermore, 4 out of 10 women had never discussed their risk for breast cancer with their physician. The findings were summarized by an excerpt from the Hughes (2013) study:

> Patients must have a better understanding of their personal risk. Study findings should help refocus educational efforts because increased knowledge of breast cancer risk will enable providers to tailor an individual's medical treatment plan.
>
> Women should be aware of their breast cancer risk number, just as they know their blood pressure, cholesterol and BMI numbers (para. 10).

Statistics obtained from the ACS (2013a) reveal that African American women suffer significantly more mortality as a result of breast cancer than European American women, even though the occurrence of breast cancer is higher in European American women. Moreover, the gap continues to widen (Howlader et al., 2013). Five-year, cause-specific breast cancer survival rates from 2003 to 2009 reveal that African American women have the lowest rates compared to other groups (ACS, 2013a). Low rates of cancer screening contribute to higher breast cancer mortality rates among African American women. Mortality may possibly be reduced if screening recommendations were utilized more efficiently.

As African American women are more likely to present with later-stage breast cancer, understanding the factors that contribute to delayed detection of breast cancer is important. Studies have shown that a 3-month delay in diagnosis of breast cancer is linked with increased mortality (Gullatte et al., 2010).

Early detection is important for minimizing mortality from breast cancer. If detected at an early stage, breast cancer can be controlled and treated (Sabatino et al., 2012). The U.S Preventive Services Task Force (2009) recommends mammography for breast cancer screening. Although screening has improved the detection of cancers, rates are suboptimal; 25%-30% of women in the recommended age groups have not had a recent mammogram (CDC, 2012; NCHS, 2010). The rates for regular screening examinations are lower (Rakowski, Wyn, Breen, Meissner, & Clark, 2010) and have not increased in recent years (Swan et al., 2010). Moreover, disparities in screening rates exist for underserved communities, particularly individuals with low income, low socioeconomic status, no health insurance, and no source of care (CDC, 2012; Swan et al., 2010).

Numerous cognitive and psychosocial factors are associated with breast cancer screening. Accordingly, behavioral interventions have been designed to promote screening among women and minimize the number of advanced stage tumors. Nevertheless, barriers to breast cancer screening are related to age, income, culture, education, knowledge, language barriers, occupation, and immigration condition (Ahmadian & Samah, 2013).

Effective programs should incorporate participation from the community, utilization of social networks and trusted social organizations, and consider cultural competence in order to reduce disparities in cancer morbidity and mortality among African American women and other ethnic groups (Ahmadian & Samah, 2013). Numerous barriers impede African American women from undergoing breast cancer screening to safeguard themselves, improve their lifestyle, and enhance their chances of survival (Deavenport et al., 2011; Todd & Stuifbergen, 2012; Young, Schwartz, & Booza, 2011) Cognitive efforts by communities and physicians are required to eliminate prevailing barriers and provide underserved African American women with opportunities for breast cancer screening (Sabatino et al.; 2012; Todd & Stuifbergen, 2012).

Conceptual Foundation

An appropriate conceptual foundation for this study is one that elucidates the way health endorsement is conceptualized and promotes the sharing of thoughts, language, and concepts between practitioners and researchers (Pasick & Burke, 2008). The theoretical foundation should propose determinants of behavioral change that can be assessed and provide a means for classifying the target population. The theoretical foundation influences the choice of intercession, predicts the expected outcomes of the intervention, suggests elements that may influence the results, and suggests strategies for improving outcomes (Pasick & Burke, 2008). The selection of a framework for an intervention is related to the number of behavioral factors, the target population, and the study environment. Theories and models represent useful tools for the development of intervention programs for health promotion (Pasick & Burke, 2008).

An appropriate theoretical foundation for this study is one that elucidates the way health endorsement is conceptualized and promotes the sharing of thoughts, language, and concepts between practitioners and researchers (Pasick & Burke, 2008). The theoretical foundation should propose determinants of behavioral change that can be assessed and provide a means for classifying the target population.

The conceptual foundation influences the choice of intercession, predicts the expected outcomes of the intervention, suggests elements that may influence the results, and suggests strategies for improving outcomes (Pasick & Burke, 2008). The selection of a framework for an intervention is related to the number of behavioral factors, the target population, and the study environment.

Many breast cancer intervention plans have been developed to improve screening adherence, informed by various socio-cognitive theories of health. The most often-used theories in regard to promotion of mammography screening are: the health belief model (Hochbaum, 1958; Rosenstock, 1960), transtheoretical model (Prochaska, 1991; Prochaska, Redding, Harlow, Rossi, & Velcier, 1994), the theory of planned behavior (Ajzen, Brown, & Carvajal, 2004), social cognitive theory (Bandura & Adams, 1977), social support theory (House, Umberson, & Landis, 1998) and the PRECEDE-PROCEED model (Green & Kreuter, 2005). According to Ahmadian and Samah (2013), the health belief model is most closely associated with breast cancer screening behaviors as this theoretical model takes into account interactions between benefits and barriers that play a vital role in health seeking behavior.

The theoretical framework for this study is the BMHSU (Andersen, 1995). This model was developed in the late 1960s to enhance understanding how and why families use health services (Andersen, 1995). The model posits that the use of health services by an individual is partly determined by predisposing, enabling, and need-related factors (Manski et al., 2013).

The model proposed the use of health services against some illnesses, assessment of individual's health behavior, and health service utilization. Andersen's framework determined that healthcare is influenced by the individual's predisposition to seek services, factors that promote the use of service, the need for medical attention, and environmental (Andersen, 1995). The dependent variables are customer satisfaction with healthcare use and various dimensions of healthcare utilization (Andersen, 1995). The health behavior model defines actual use of health services as the dependent variables or health outcome. The dependent variables could measure purpose of visit, the type of service sought, site at which service was administered, and the time interval between last visits (Andersen. 1995). In later models (Andersen, 2008), the health outcome variables incorporated consumer satisfaction, which was intended to examine the rising health care cost and the subsequent need to substantiate the continuing existence of certain health care centers. Availability of service, convenience, financial options, quality of service, and provider characteristics were treated as indicators of consumer satisfaction (Andersen, 1995).

Key Variables and Concepts

African American women are diagnosed at later stages of breast cancer and lesser 5-year survival rates are noted when compared to European American women (ACS, 2011). Breast cancer is emerging as an increasingly critical public health concern among African American women.

Ability of culturally effective interventions to improve screening rates and reduce mortality depend on obtaining accurate information about barriers to screening in this population (ACS, 2011; Cancer Research UK, 2010). The ACS screening guidelines suggest that women aged 40 years and above with average risk for breast cancer should have yearly mammograms, and there is no specific upper age limit when breast screening through mammography should be terminated. Women aged 20 years and above should undergo a three-stage test procedure, namely BSE, CBE, and mammography (ACS, 2013c). First, BSE should be performed on a regular basis, and women should be aware of the advantages and limitations of BSE. New breast symptoms should be reported to a health care professional. Next women between the ages of 20 and 30 years should undergo periodic CBE, at least once every 3 years, while women over age 40 should receive at least one CBE every year (ACS, 2013c).

Physicians and the health care systems play an important role in facilitating individual's participation in cancer screening and in providing valuable care. Targeted intervention strategies must be devised to improve cancer screening rates (ACS, 2013c).

Young et al. (2011) studied 178 African American women, aged 40 years and above, who resided in high cancer-risk areas and identified personal, structural, and clinical barriers to obtaining mammograms. Limiting barriers to mammograms included the level of education of the patient and communication skills, individual barriers included lack of knowledge and trust, and structural barriers included lack of insurance, care providers and facilities (Young et al.; 2011). Efforts by medical practitioners to minimize medical barriers to mammography screening in African American women should focus on increased and improved communication between physician and patient and education related to breast cancer knowledge to address fears around mammography (Young, Schwartz, & Booza, 2011).

Hardin (2012) found that over 40% of fears related to mammography were associated with anxiety related to the outcome. Over 30% of fears related to mammography were in regard to pain and getting retested. Other fears included exposure of the body, monetary factors, radiation, and lack of or limited knowledge about the procedure.

Gierisch et al. (2009) reported that the foremost reasons for underutilization of mammography were cost and distance and Cardarelli et al. (2013) identified economic and structural barriers associated with breast cancer screening. The fee for mammography is one of the leading factors that contribute to low rates of breast cancer screening through mammography. Poor awareness, lack of mammography sites, and lack of transportation to mammography sites are other barriers to mammography screening. Studies have also shown that decreased barriers are associated with increased benefits that are directly related to enhance screening.

Ahmadian and Samah (2011), in a survey of Iranian women, found that high levels of distress are associated with nonadherence to mammography screening guidelines. Cancer screening behaviors directly influence prevention of breast cancer, timely detection, incidence rates, diagnosis, and treatment and after treatment effect, life value, and survival for African American women. Three major types of cancer screening behaviors have been identified: (a) poverty and low socioeconomic status, (b) social injustice, and (c) culture (Conway-Phillips & Janusek, 2014; Conway-Phillips & Millon-Underwood, 2009). These will be discussed in the following sections.

Barriers Associated with Poverty and Low Socioeconomic Status

Poverty is the primary social factor involved in health disparities. Poverty directly correlates with low socioeconomic status and is related to the reduced rates of breast cancer screening among these populations. (U.S. Department of Education, National Center for Educational Statistics, 2008). Socioeconomic status is the combined total measure of the economic and social position of an individual or family in relation to others. The measure includes income, education, and occupation (U.S. Department of Education, National Center for Educational Statistics, 2008).

Low screening rates may result in higher incidences of late-stage diagnosis. Such cases receive inadequate treatment, which is followed by higher mortality rates (Ahmed, Winter, Albatineh, & Haber, 2012). As most African Americans live in conditions of poverty, this factor has emerged as the chief barrier to breast cancer screening behavior. Financial issues influence access to health care through factors such as insurance status, transportation to screening sites, loss of job-related income (taking unpaid time off to attend screening sites), and childcare (Ahmed et al., 2012). These factors affect African Americans disproportionately since more African Americans live in poverty compared to European Americans (Ahmed et al., 2012).

Lack of Primary Care

Lack of a primary care physician also serves as a barrier to breast cancer screening and follow up. Poverty prevents women from having a regular care provider who can provide CBE and mammography referrals. (ACS, Cancer Action Network, 2009). Studies reveal that individuals that have regular, preferred and trusted care provider are two times as likely to undergo mammography screening in comparison with women without a primary care provider, and those who visit for mammography are more likely to revisit. Due to poverty, African American women remain underserved and fail to draw benefits from access to primary care (ACS, Cancer Action Network, 2009).

Geographical Distribution of Care Facilities

African Americans tend to live in geographical areas that lack physicians and clinics, which make breast cancer screening, diagnosis, and treatment more difficult (Todd & Stuifbergen, 2012). An African American woman who wishes to be screened for breast cancer may be required to travel lengthy distances with extended waiting times. Elongated travel time, civic transportation hassles, and scheduling procedures at awkward hours have been described as chief factors that prevent breast cancer healthy behaviors among African American women (Todd & Stuifbergen, 2012).

Competing Priorities

Poverty prevents African American women from setting priorities for health and taking steps to prevent breast cancer through screening activities. African American women have more demanding survival requirements that encompass food, clothing, shelter, and safety (Hatcher-Keller, Rayens, Dignan, Schoenberg, & Allison 2013). In addition, many

African American women work on an hourly basis and do not get paid for time off to attend breast cancer screening facilities. Having to focus more attention on safety and survival, African American women may not be able to devote sufficient attention to breast cancer screening as they are focusing more on primary needs (Hatcher-Keller et al., 2013; Rahman et al., 2009).

Comorbidity

Comorbidity explains racial disparities that prevail in breast cancer treatment and mortality. Conditions of comorbidity include hypertension, cardiovascular disease, diabetes, and respiratory disease, which are more rampant among African American women than in European American women. Poor patients are unable to adhere to treatment and post-treatment regimes and, in the case of multiple comorbidities, it becomes difficult for African American women to pay attention to any one particular disease condition (Simonds, Colditz, Rudd, & Sequest, 2011).

Health insurance

Inappropriate health insurance due to poverty is a factor in racial health disparities. Low wages force African American women to either remain uninsured or to use public insurance such as Medicaid. Uninsured and underinsured women are usually reluctant to opt for breast cancer screening and, as a result, they are more likely to present with late-stage detection of breast cancer (Hoffman et al., 2011).

Privately insured women present at earlier stages compared to publicly insured women, and publicly insured women present at earlier stages than uninsured women (Hoffman et al., 2011; Komenaka et al., 2010).

Lack of Knowledge and Information

A poor financial situation is directly proportional to poor education and understanding about breast cancer screening and the importance of early detection and treatment. Compared to European Americans, African Americans are less likely to understand the guidelines and recommendations of the ACS. Poverty also contributes to poor dietary habits among African Americans. They consume more fats and fewer fruits and vegetables (Sheppard et al., 2013).

Risk-promoting lifestyles

Poverty is related to high-risk lifestyles that include poor nutrition, lack or inadequate physical activity, and postmenopausal obesity, which are predisposing factors for breast cancer. African American women are more prone to be obese as they eat a high-fat diet and few fruits and vegetables (Gehlert & Coleman, 2010). African American residential areas are devoid of open spaces, parks, and sidewalks, so they have few chances to exercise (Gehlert & Coleman, 2010; Menashe, Anderson, Jatoi, & Rosenberg, 2009). Moreover, African American women residing in urban areas experience increased risks in terms of safety, which contributes to a risk-promoting lifestyle as the safety issues prevent them from participating in outdoor physical exercises.

Provider and System-level Factors

Poverty among African American women has a negative impact on the behavior and attitude of health care providers and access to health services (Conway-Phillips & Janusek, 2014).

Physicians who are less qualified are more likely to serve communities of low socioeconomic status, which lowers the probability of asking African American women to participate in breast cancer screening procedures such as mammography (Alexandraki & Mooradian, 2010).

Barriers Related to Culture

Cultural factors promote cultural and racial disparities in breast cancer screening, detection, treatment, adherence to treatment regimens, and mortality. Cultural beliefs about breast cancer and sharing among African Americans play a vital role in breast cancer screening behaviors (Conway-Phillips & Janusek, 2014).

Perceived Susceptibility to Breast Cancer

African American women tend to consider their normal selves to be at low risk for developing breast cancer and therefore do not feel the need for mammograms. This low-risk perception and participation in screening results in delays in seeking treatment for breast cancer. In addition, cultural norms prevent African American women from discussing breast cancer and thus diminish the salience of breast cancer screening (Umezawa et al., 2012).

Cultural convictions and thoughts

European American and African American women possess different viewpoint about breast cancer. African American women are of the opinion that a small, non-painful lump in the breast may not be cancerous, and that BSE is the best method for early onset detection of breast cancer. Moreover, there persists a culture-specific apprehension linked to breast cancer (Breast Care Site, 2009; Kingsley, 2010). Fears related to emotional distress, uneasiness, embarrassment, and radiation contribute to low rates of screening by mammography. These apprehensions may lead to delayed breast cancer detection. African American women have low confidence in Western medicine and believe that cutting into cancerous breast tissue may expose it to air and promote its spread (Adams et al., 2009; Breast Care Site, 2009; Kingsley, 2010).

Medical Mistrust

African American women lack trust in the western system of medicine. They are rigid about their decisions to seek medical attention and interactions with health care providers (Greer-Williams et al., 2014; Masi & Gehlert, 2009). For example, the medical mistrust that the Tuskegee syphilis tragedy caused continues to affect African Americans in their decision to accept medical care. The Tuskegee experiment was initiated by the U.S. Public Health Service (PHS) in 1932 and lasted through 1972. The experiment was designed to monitor the health outcome of syphilis on 400 black men in Tuskegee, Alabama (Bates & Harris, 2004). These men were discriminated against and were not treated for syphilis despite the invention of penicillin; rather, they were given placebo and lied to that they were being treated. As a result, many of the men died. Unfortunately, the memory of this study remains a barrier for public trust (Bates & Harris, 2004).

Barriers Related to Social Injustice

Racial prejudice may contribute to disparities in mammography referrals between African American and European American women. African Americans frequently state lack of health care provider or physician referral as the reason for not pursuing breast cancer screening (Bowen et al., 2013). Physicians, who are mostly European American rate African American patients as less educated, less intellectual, and more inclined to abuse drugs hence leading to lesser referral rates. These factors impede breast cancer screening for African American women, which contributes to high rates of mortality (Bowen et al., 2013; Kingsley, 2010).

Cardarelli et al. (2013) identified 15 barriers that impede breast cancer screening on the basis of interviews with underserved women. These barriers include: (a) 25% fear of cancer detection; (b) 23 % unaware of the details of the procedure; (c) around 25 % accessibility of mammogram; (d) about 5 % believed that screening for mammogram is embarrassing; (e) about <5% believed that mammogram is time consuming; (f) about 7% feared risk of exposure to radiation; (g) about 10% believed that they have more important issues than mammogram; (h) about <5% believed that there is no need for mammogram; (i) about 40% believed that affordability is an issue; (j) about 37% had transportation issues; (k) about 35% proximity to home; (l) about 6% had issues with privacy of information; (m) about 6% believed that exposing their breasts made them uncomfortable; (n) about 5% found the closeness of the x-ray staff uncomfortable; (o) about 47% reported they could not afford a mammogram and were not aware of any free mammogram. These results indicate that poor education levels among African American women are responsible for advanced stage detection, late diagnosis, and late onset of treatment of breast cancer in this population (Cardarelli et al., 2013). These factors contribute to higher cancer mortality rates compared to European American women, even though incidence rates are lower in the former group.

Rationale for Phenomenological Research

The review of literature confirmed a lack of qualitative research particularly investigating the perception of African American women in regard to their personal barriers, attitudes, and beliefs to breast cancer screening. The lack of understanding with reference to African American women perspectives necessitates a qualitative phenomenological approach. Phenomenology is a qualitative study approach that focuses on the need to study human perception of the world that the study participants personally experience (Spiegelberg, 1995). In this proposed study, the in-depth interviews of 14 African American women in an urban East Coast region will promote the phenomenological understanding of their experiences with the barriers to breast cancer prevention and screening. The emerging themes from the interviews will help answer the research questions:

RQ: What are the perceived barriers for breast cancer screening among African American Women?

Sub-RQs:

Sub-RQ1: How can awareness of breast cancer screening and prevention be promoted among African American women?

Sub-RQ2: How does stereotype and culture influence African American women's beliefs and behavior in regard to breast cancer screening and prevention?

Previous studies have been conducted using phenomenological approach in healthcare profession to understand patients' perception of their life occurrence. Subramanian, Burhan, Pallaveshi, & Rudnick (2013) conducted a study with the aim to understand the lived experience of patients with schizophrenia who were treated for auditory hallucination with Repetitive Transcranial Magnetic Stimulation. The researchers used semi-structured interviews method to collect patients' data on belief and way of thinking. Likewise, Sadala, Bruzos, Pereira, and Bucuvic (2012) used a phenomenological approach to understand the severe effect of disease on patients' health and their experience during the disease process. The result of the study confirmed the need for health care providers to acknowledge and respect patients' experiences in order to enhance positive health outcomes.

Summary and Conclusion

Breast cancer screening is the safest means to detect cancer at an early stage. Three methods for breast examination are BSE, CBE, and mammography. European American females display a greater incidence of breast cancer compared to African American women, but mortality rates from breast cancer are greater in the latter group. Such disparities in cancer incidence and mortality can be attributed to various barriers to preventative breast health care for African American women, including factors related to poverty and low socioeconomic status, social injustice, and culture.

Health care providers must bridge the prevailing gap in health care by informing African American women about breast cancer and the importance of breast examination and providing them with appropriate care and treatment. By addressing issues related to racial injustice, which is one of the key determinants of breast cancer disparities, breast cancer screening can be promoted in this underprivileged and underserved community of African American women.

Providing immediate medical coverage will increase diagnoses at earlier stages of breast cancer. By identifying and targeting geographical areas where the density of African Americans is high, and by providing funding to the African American community, timely and adequate detection could be promoted. Strategies for reformation must include provisions for health care, liberty to hourly workers so that they can seek breast cancer screening without suffering loss of pay and promoting a better understanding and self- awareness of the significance of breast cancer screening. However, more study is essential to better understand the barriers to breast cancer screening in this population and help eliminate disparities due to race and ethnicity. By addressing issues related to socioeconomic status, the association between breast cancer survival and race could be eliminated. Chapter 3 will further explain the detailed methods for this research project.

Chapter 3:
Research Method

Introduction

Reducing persistent disparities in health may offer the potential for enhancing the health status of the general population. In this qualitative study, I explored African American women's professed personal barriers, stereotype, socioeconomic status, culture, attitudes, beliefs, and how these factors influenced breast cancer screening. The goal of qualitative methodology is to clarify and offer an insight on multifaceted psychosocial matters and is a research design of choice in answering many humanistic why and how questions (Marshall, 1996).

Breast cancer is considered a major cancer in females and among the main causes of cancer mortality amongst women in the United States (ACS, 2011; Jemal et al., 2005). Although immense progress has been made in screening procedures and mammography practices for the general population, lesser screening rates are seen in various female subgroups (ACS, 2011; U.S. Department of Health and Human Services, CDC [CDC], 2013). Tumors are commonly detected and diagnosed among ethnic minority communities at an advanced stage. Without exploring individual professed barriers to breast cancer screening amid African American women, breast cancer will continue to be one of the causes of mortality in African American women (American Cancer Society, Surveillance Research, 2011). In this chapter, I describe the qualitative research paradigm and rationale for this study of African American women.

In addition, I describe the process for this study, which includes the description of the study participants, inclusion criteria, and the role of the researcher credibility, and issues of trustworthiness for the study. This chapter also includes an explanation of the data collection, how the data will be collected and analyzed, biases and threats to data quality.

Research Design and Rationale

I explored individual barriers to breast cancer screening among African American women 40 years and older. According to ACS recommendations, at the age of 40, all three protocols of BSE, CBE and mammography need to be followed per guideline. However, ACS recommends beginning BSE at 20 years of age. The decision to base this study on women aged 40 years and older was based on ACS recommendation and it is also the age recommended for screening by most cancer control programs (Patton, 2002). Understanding this phenomenon may help healthcare providers improve services that may bridge the gap in healthcare disparity.

Shank (2006) defined qualitative research as a form of systematic empirical inquiry into meaning (p. 4). The use of qualitative research allowed me as the researcher to plan an intentional approach to studying the complexities of situations, experiences, or phenomena. Such qualitative inquiry included three tenets: the researcher matters, the inquiry into meaning is in service of understanding, and qualitative inquiry embraces new ways of looking at the world (Shank, 2006, p. 10)

Using qualitative approach ensured reporting the findings of the study as obtained directly from the study participants and not subjected to any manipulation of variables as expected in quantitative studies (Patton, 2002). Another rationale for choosing qualitative methodology over quantitative is that the information gathered from the participants is reflective of the study participants' viewpoint about the human race (Patton, 2002). Spiegelberg (1995) described six essential uses of phenomenology approach namely, descriptive phenomenology, essential phenomenology, phenomenology of appearances, constitutive phenomenology, reductive phenomenology and hermeneutic (Interpretative) phenomenology (p. 57). Of the six mentioned approaches above, Interpretative phenomenology approach (IPA) formed the basis of this study as this approach provides understanding of participants' personal experience (Spiegelberg, 1995). According to Cresswell, (2007) a phenomenology provides a deep understanding of a phenomenon as experienced by several individuals.

Interpretative phenomenology approach enabled me gather comprehensive perspective on how African American women understood and viewed breast cancer screening, professed personal barriers, stereotype, socio-economic status, culture, attitudes, beliefs, and how these factors influenced their breast cancer screening (Smith, 2004) IPA produces a universal claim or principle from observed instance (inductive), as well as paying close attention to particular cases and the distinctive characteristics or ability of people, rather than on extensive generalizations in relation to human behavior which is characterized by the distinctiveness of each case (idiographic), IPA is also interrogative and involves questioning or seeming to question somebody or something (Smith, 2004). IPA is flexible and evolves collection of factual information from individuals unlike trying to validate detailed hypotheses. IPA begins with research questions that tend to find meaning to specific phenomena of study (Smith, 2004).

Each case was reviewed individually and then the information gathered examined closely, in order to have more understanding or draw conclusions from it until all cases in the study are explored. Discovery of the common themes in all the cases were determined through cross examination. Personal perspectives were learned in addition to those. Additionally, individual accounts are revealed as well as those evident across all cases (Smith, 2004). IPA is probing as it results in comprehensive examination of observable facts and the findings contribute to existing literature. I considered IPA the most suitable qualitative methodological design for my study because it provided me the outmost opportunity to carry out an expansive analysis of the study participants' expression and meaning influencing their professed factors affecting breast cancer screening. IPA also gave me the opportunity to obtain first-hand information and understanding about each participant's world. In addition, "the only way for us to really know what another person experience is to experience the phenomenon as directly as possible for ourselves" (Patton 2002, p. 106). Patton realized the importance of study methodology and indicated that observing participants and thorough interview study method are the ways to better understand the culture of those participants.

In conclusion, I hope that the phenomenology research method chosen would provide insight into the individual experiences of African American women professed personal barriers that may influence breast cancer screening. Hopefully, this will help healthcare providers improve on healthcare services that may bridge the gap in healthcare disparity

Role of the Researcher

In qualitative study, the researcher is identified as the key instrument for data collection (Draper & Swift, 2011), and a researcher is obligated to have an effective listening ability, honest, pleasant, flexible, and non-judgmental. Qualitative study has many varieties of approaches hence gives the researcher many options about data collection, and serves as a form of content analysis ranging from observational phenomenological psychology to complex interpretation of context depending on the data source (Draper & Swift, 2011). In my study, I served as the main instrument for data collection to ensure that I identified, comprehended what I needed to study, and how to achieve my goal. My role included: finding my study site and study participants. It was important that I initiated a friendly relationship that gave me the opportunity to understand and showed the study participants that I valued and shared their concerns from my initial contact with the leaders of the community. This approach contributed to my gaining access to the participant's story (Dickson-Swift, James, Kippen, & Liamputton, 2007). My roles also included maintaining good interpersonal relationship with the participants hence facilitated co-operation, obtained more information, and made them felt at ease during and after the interview process (Glesne, 2011). To promote positive and healthy relationship, I ensured that each participant clarified any concerns they had before interview, and the participants had the advantage to evaluate the interview questions prior to the planned interview. I began each individual interview by appreciating the participant's willingness to assist in my study; I introduced the research study to each participant and explained to them that they are welcome any time to decline answering any questions or exit from the interview process whenever they wanted. Privacy is a vital factor in research. As a result, appropriate measures were implemented to ascertain the confidentiality of all study participants.

To protect the identity of the participants, all names were coded; for example P1 for participant 1, the participants' information were stored electronically on a computer with secured password and in a locked filling cabinet, and the tape recordings were well protected and the raw data will be kept for a minimum of five years With measures in place to protect the participants, they were willing to cooperate with me more as they were assured that confidentiality is maintained at all times. It was also my role to empower the participants through providing them with adequate information of the research process and the measures taken to protect their human rights by fulfilling the requirement of the Institutional Review Board (IRB) and obtained permission for the study (Creswell, 2009). My responsibility as the researcher in this study was to play the role of the observer and the interviewer to find answers to the inquiry to be investigated. Probing is a productive tool to use by a researcher as it encourages interviewees to furnish the interviewer with comprehensive or specific answer to a given question. Hence allows the interviewer to attain the specific information on which the research study is centered.

To prevent bias towards the participants' responses to the interview questions, I had an open mind at all times. Specific probing techniques that helped me to prevent biases included the use of open-ended questions, tracking, clarification, and reflective summary (Patton, 2002). Open-ended questions provided interviewees with full opportunity to communicate their feelings, and allowed participants to answer questions in the manner they wanted using their own words (Patton, 2002). Tracking is the involvement of the interviewer by showing interest in the interviewee, encourages the interviewee to speak and observes all verbal and non-verbal conversation. Through clarification, I got more understanding of the interviewee's responses, for example what factors in your opinion would better enhance your experience and/or utilization of breast cancer screening? Reflective summary is the ability of the interviewer to repeat the ideas, opinions and feelings of interviewees correctly in his/her own words.

Methodology

Participant Selection Logic

The study participants were recruited from a local church in an urban east coast region using purposeful sampling after IRB approval. The participants were African American women aged 40 years and older until a point of saturation was reached (Walker, 2012). To obtain sample size representative of the perception of participants, at minimum 14 participants was realistic. I used a purposeful sampling method. Sample inclusion criteria included (a) African American females 40 years of age or older (b) no previous or present diagnosis of breast cancer (c) ability to communicate in English Language effectively (d) participants were African American women who were willing to share their professed personal barriers, stereotype, socio-economic status, culture, attitudes, beliefs, and how these factors influenced breast cancer screening. Getting participants was not as difficult as thought owing to the sensitivity of the proposed study.

In meeting with the gatekeepers of the community which are the people at the research sites known to have the capability to provide access to the site and thereby allow the study to proceed (Creswell, 2009); I provided them with the information on the nature of the intended study. The pre-interview preparation also included getting in contact with the volunteers and presenting the details of the study. During the meeting, I informed the individuals that I will be posting fliers at the information boards which will explain my intention, their rights and if they believe they meet the inclusion criteria to contact me. (Copy of the flyer can be found in Appendix C). This ensured that the potential participants were the ones to identify themselves as (a) African American females 40 years of age or older (b) no previous or present diagnosis of breast cancer (c) ability to communicate in English Language effectively and would permit interested individuals to read my inclusion criteria and then identify themselves to me as possible participants (d) participants will be women who are willing to share their professed personal barriers, stereotype, socio-economic status, culture, attitudes, beliefs, and how these factors may influence breast cancer screening. I posted flyers (Appendix C) in the participants' local church. Interested women contacted me to initiate the interview procedure.

Measures

The purpose of this study was to understand African American women's professed personal barriers, stereotype, socioeconomic status, culture, attitudes, beliefs, and how these factors may influence breast cancer screening. The research questions that helped me to better understand their experiences contained one central question and two sub-questions.

RQ: What are the perceived barriers for breast cancer screening among African American Women?

Sub-RQs

Sub-RQ1: How can awareness of breast cancer screening and prevention be promoted among African American women?

Sub-RQ2: How does stereotype and culture influence African American women's beliefs and behavior in regard to breast cancer screening and prevention?

Ethical Protection of Participants

I obtained Institutional Review Board approval from Walden University on 05-12-15 and IRB# 0231648. The study participants were African American volunteers who had the right either to be or not to be involved in the study. There were minimal risks associated with participating in this study with interview questions that may be considered personal or private. I ensured the anonymity of the participants and offered them the choice of opting out at any time. No participant experienced harm or difficulty from volunteering in my study. All participants filled out individual consent forms and their confidentiality was protected. Sample copies of the document for consent to audiotape and confidentiality statement can be found in Appendix A. Any identifying information of the participants from transcripts were removed prior to data validation. All research materials such as transcripts, files and audiotapes are securely preserved in a protected cupboard in my office. Only the researcher will have access to research information.

Procedures for Recruitment and Participation

Procedure for recruitment and participation for the intended study started upon approval by IRB. The following measures were adhered to during the process of recruiting study participants, data collection, data examination, and validation of findings.

1. I identified a church in an urban East Coast region as the site for my interview.

2. I found/identified the gatekeeper of the community.

3. I approached the gatekeeper of the community, and introduced myself to the individual as a Walden University student who was requesting to conduct my research study interview in their community.

4. The gatekeeper approved of my intention, and I sent a letter via email to the gatekeeper with information about my study, inclusion criteria and appeal for backing in allowing me to use their facility to interview the self-identified individuals who were willing to participate in my study. I discussed my need to have a Letter of Cooperation from the gatekeeper and requested the individual's preference either to provide me with the letter before or after IRB approval. The gatekeeper provided me with a Letter of Cooperation prior to IRB approval.

5. I requested to have about10-15 minutes to introduce myself to the potential participants during one of their weekly

sessions at which time I informed the individuals that I would be posting fliers at their information boards which would explain my intention and their rights. They were informed that if they believed that they met the inclusion criteria, they were to contact me. (Copy of the flyer can be found in Appendix C). This approach was to ensure that the potential participants were the ones to identify themselves as African American women 18 – 45 years old. This would permit interested individuals to read my inclusion criteria and then identify themselves to me as possible participants.

6. I formalized the intention of the potential volunteers who contacted me. I thanked each potential participant for their intention to participate in my study.

7. I scheduled a face-to-face meeting with self-identified participants and clarified any concerns or questions. During this meeting, I showed the individuals a copy of the IRB approval certificate to reassure the participants that my study was approved by my school. The potential participants were required to sign and date the consent form. I gave the consent form to each participant. I fully explained the contents of the consent form and their concerns were addressed. Participants were given the consent form to take home and I collected the forms at each individual's interview.

8. I requested a day for the interview and worked around each potential participant's schedule. The interview included

asking questions listed in Appendix B, Interview Protocol, which were developed by me to aid and answer the research questions. The interviews were scheduled at the convenience of the study participant during one hour time blocks in a private room where confidentiality was observed and identity kept private. All interviews were audio-recorded. I used observation notes which provided a secondary data source.

To promote positive and healthy relationship, I ensured that each participant expressed any concerns they had before the interview, and the participants had the advantage of evaluating the interview questions prior to the planned interview. I began each individual interview by appreciating the participant's willingness to assist in my study; I introduced the research study to each participant and explained to them that they were welcome any time to decline answering any questions or exit from the interview process whenever they wanted.

9. A second interview was scheduled two weeks after the interview. This was to allow me time to transcribe the audiotapes verbatim and analyze the text data.

Instrumentation

I recruited 14 African American women aged 40 years and older. I anticipated saturation would be met after conducting at least 14-16 interviews. Saturation occurred when all 21 questions had been totally explored in detail and no new themes were gained from additional interviews (Walker, 2012). Studies have recommended a certain acceptable sample size for qualitative research with participants' number ranging from five to 50 participants (Mason, 2010). I estimated that a starting sample of 14 would be adequate and to which to include more participants if needed.

The interviews were scheduled at the convenience of the study participant during 1 hour time blocks in a private room where confidentiality and identity were kept private. All interviews were audio-recorded. Observation notes provided a secondary data source. Interview questions were directed towards answering the research questions based upon the literature review in Chapter 2 and the assumption that the participants shared their professed barriers on breast cancer screening and prevention. Study participants were recruited and interviewed until saturation of the data was met. A pilot study was conducted. I contacted self-identified participants in an urban east coast region. An invitation to participate was made during a meeting that was organized by the gatekeeper. At the meeting, I informed the individuals that I will be posting fliers at their information boards which would explain my intention, their rights and whether they believed they met the inclusion criteria to contact me. During the meeting, I informed the individuals that I would be posting fliers at the information boards which would explain my intention, their rights and if they believe they met the inclusion criteria to contact me. (Copy of the flyer can be found in

Appendix C). This was to ensure that the potential participants were the ones to identify themselves as (a) African American females 40 years of age or older (b) having no previous or present diagnosis of breast cancer (c) being able to communicate in English Language effectively and permit interested individuals to read my inclusion criteria and then identify themselves to me as possible participants (d) women who were willing to share their professed personal barriers, stereotype, socio-economic status, culture, attitudes, beliefs, and how these factors may influence breast cancer screening.

Pilot Study Procedures

A pilot study was conducted with one known volunteer practitioner. The rationale of the pilot study was to ensure that the interview questions would provide information that would answer the research questions. The pilot study was conducted in the same location as the actual study participant interviews. Administering a pilot study helped to eliminate mechanical or planning and management problems that may occur during the actual interviews. The pilot study gave me the opportunity to practice audio-recording, my interview techniques which included, establishing good rapport through a professional self-introduction to the participants, explanation of the informed consent, conducting and closing techniques of open-ended interview. The data collected during the pilot study is not included in the final data analysis.

Exiting the Study

Study participants were informed that their participation was completely voluntary, and they had the option to opt out at any time they wished to do so.

Data Analysis Plan

Understanding participants' personal and social worlds, particularly how participants make sense of their world, can be better understood through interpretive phenomenological analysis (Smith & Osborn, 2003). The aim of interpretive approach is to recognize the significance of the content and complexity of those meanings. As a result, the primary nature of IPA research is for researchers to find meaning to the participants' experience (Patton, 2002; Smith, 2004). To aid this understanding, it is recommended that immediately after an interview; a researcher should reflect and interpret the study findings (Feldman, 1981; Seidman, 2006). After the interview, I reflected on the process, transcribed and analyzed the data I collected by implementing IPA method. In order to conduct a thorough analysis, I listened, understood each interview case one at a time until all cases were explored prior to analysis. To analyze the cases thoroughly and develop a theme, I used Smith, Jarman, and Osborn (1999) six step analytical process.

The process is analyzed in the figure below.

Figure 1 The Six-Step analytical process

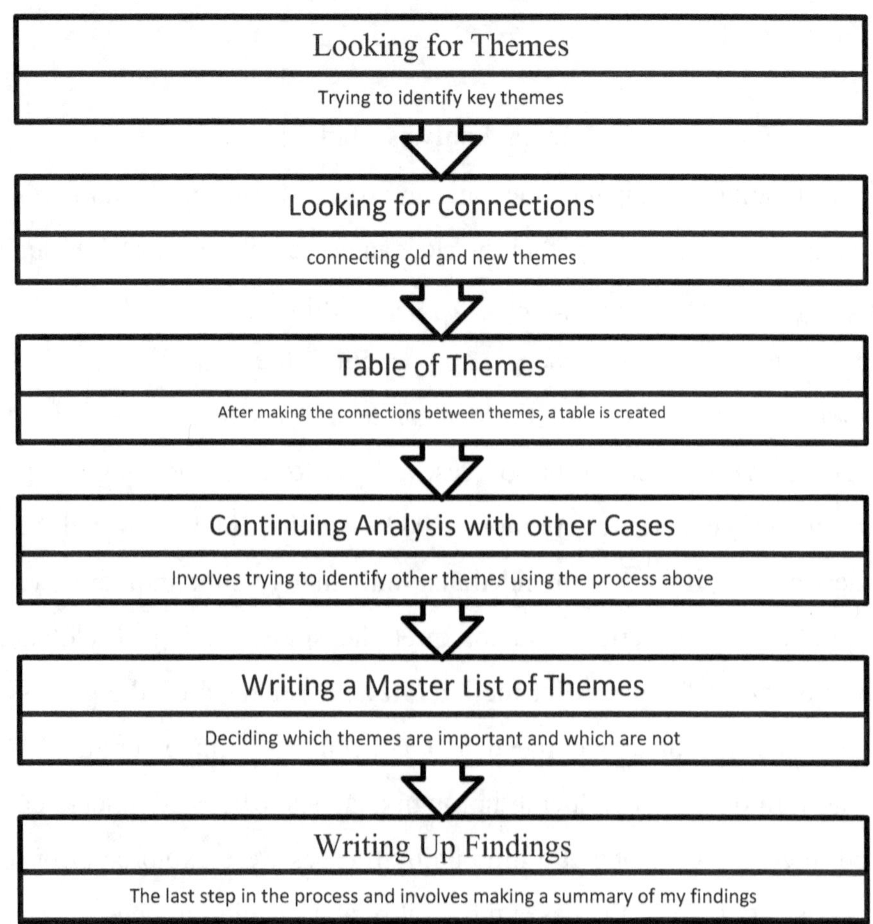

Table 1: The Six-Step Analytical Process

Step	Approach
Step 1: Looking for themes	I started my analysis by reading the initial case which were documented in a two-column arrangement to ensure that interpretive and reflection records of each interview are documented separately. This approach limited my preconceived notion and to maintain integrity of the volunteers' exclusive responses with this phenomenon (Smith et al., 1999). While I read each case, new understanding of the participants' experience were acknowledged and documented into the column on the transcription. I was able to establish emerging themes from the notes and then documented in the column of main themes (Collingridge & Grant, 2008; Smith et al., 1999). Following documentation of all notes, I imported transcripts to NVivo to support and aid with my data analysis. During this process of

	looking for themes, I ensured that I treated each transcript as a possible data and no attempt was made to alter, discard or exclude any information from the document.
Step 2: Looking for connection	I created a listing of new themes and made a connection between the old and the new themes. As themes were being arranged into a group, I compared the result with the original record to note the correlation (Smith & Osborn, 2003). The rationale of step 2 was to have some sort of arrangement of the themes that were compiled from the participants' responses (Smith et al., 1999).
Step 3: Producing a table of theme	According to Smith and Osborn (2003), in compiling a table of themes, some unconnected information to the other themes should be set aside if such information cannot be established by data collected in the transcripts. I then organized the themes into a table and named them accordingly.

Step 4: Continuing the analysis with other cases	I continued with the analysis of other participants' responses (P1-P14) to the interview questions utilizing the steps above to further generate my record of themes
Step 5: Creating a master list of themes	After gathering all the themes from each case, I then concluded on which themes will be listed on the master list of themes. The decision to place a theme on the master list was determined by the significance of the text in support of the theme.
Step 6: Writing up findings	I transferred the information on the master theme list into a comprehensive report which was the study participants' responses during my interview. It is required that the raw data is kept secure for a minimum of five years after which the data will be thoroughly and completely destroyed in such a way that information cannot be extracted by process of shredding

and secure destruction of all written records.

Issues of Trustworthiness

Trustworthiness is vital in qualitative study, and it ascertains the validity and reliability of qualitative research (European American, Oelke, & Friesen, 2012). Qualitative research is trustworthy when it is the accurate representation of the study participants' experiences. Trustworthiness ascertains the validity and reliability of qualitative research (European American et al., 2012). To demonstrate trustworthiness in my study, I ensured that the experiences of the participants were accurately represented. Trustworthiness of data in method triangulation was demonstrated. As a result, I paid attention to and confirmed all information gathered and examined the evidence from them to create a logical justification of the underlying themes.

Four criteria were used to measure trustworthiness of data (European American et al., 2012): credibility, dependability, transferability and confirmability.

Credibility

Credibility is maintained when participants are able to identify their own experiences from researcher reported research findings as their own experiences (King & Horrocks, 2010). To ensure credibility, I ensured that participants were identified and described accurately. I completed member checks in which my interpretations and conclusions of each interview case could be tested with each study participant from whom the data were originally collected. I demonstrated triangulation by paying attention to and confirmation of information discovery.

Triangulation is a qualitative approach that relies on several technique or information sources (Glesne, 2011). My information resources included participants' experiences gathered through interviews, literature, and documented information. A researcher has to be mindful of study biases. As a result, I put aside what I already knew which I implemented at all times during my research process and also handled each phase of my study with care (Creswell, 2009). Reviewing the phenomenon under study to evade bias and advance with the research process with a receptive mind was also implemented. I also maintained rigor in the process of collecting my data by continuing the documentation of recruitment, collection data of techniques, progressive data examination, and other data relevant to the study (Creswell, 2009)

Transferability

Transferability is the likelihood of a particular study result having similar interpretation by others when transferred to another setting in similar situations (Crosby, DiClemente, & Salazar, 2006). I maintained transferability by ensuring that I described and documented precisely the study participants' perspective and the statements central to the research.

Dependability

Dependability is related to consistency of findings, whereby researchers from any other setting will have the same study result when a new study is conducted with the same participants (Crosby et al., 2006; Creswell, 2009). Appropriate strategies to establish dependability included use of audit trails and triangulation. The rationale was to assess the correctness and assess whether or not the findings, interpretations and conclusions were in accordance with the data collected.

Confirmability

Confirmability is another standard for measuring the trustworthiness of qualitative research. Confirmability is the level to which the research findings are true to the study participants' view and not influenced by researcher's bias or analysis (Lincoln & Guba, 1985). To enhance confirmability, I ensured to interpret and conclude research findings solely from data collected. I was mindful to observe rather than dictate the direction of the interviews and asked the study participants for clarification of any unfamiliar words.

Summary

This chapter explored the methods and procedures for my study of African American women's professed personal barriers, stereotype, socio-economic status, culture, attitudes, beliefs, and how these factors may influence breast cancer screening. Other main points explored in this chapter included me, the researcher as the main instrument for data collection, and ethical issues in data collection and sampling techniques.

Chapter 4 covers results of the pilot study, setting, demographics of participants, the data analysis, and results.

Chapter 4:
Results

Introduction

The purpose of this qualitative, phenomenological study was to explore individual barriers to breast cancer screening among 40 years and older African American women to better understand why breast cancer continues to be one of the principal sources of mortality among African American women. In addition, the purposes included identifying barriers to preventive screening for breast cancer among African American women and to explore the influence of personal barriers, stereotypes, socioeconomic status, culture, attitudes, and beliefs on the behavior of African American women in regard to breast cancer screening.

The research questions contained one central question and two sub questions. Central RQ: What are the perceived barriers for breast cancer screening among African American Women? Sub-RQ1: How can awareness of breast cancer screening and prevention be promoted among African American women? Sub-RQ2: How does stereotype and culture influence African American women's beliefs and behavior in regard to breast cancer screening and prevention?

The conceptual framework for this study was the behavioral model of health services use which affirmed that the use of health services by an individual is partly determined by predisposing, enabling, and need factors. In this chapter, I will present the results of interviews with 14 African American women. The interviews were conducted between May and June 2015. In this chapter, I will also describe the participant demographics, data collection procedure, the pilot study, data analysis and relevant themes, and quality of data.

Pilot Study

After gaining Walden University IRB approval, I completed a pilot study with one volunteer, a 62-year-old African American woman. This was done one week prior to the start of actual data collection. The purpose of the pilot study was to ensure that the interview questions provided data that would answer the research questions, to help to eliminate mechanical or planning and management problems that could occur during the interviews, and to ensure a meaningful interview process. The volunteer met all the inclusion criteria for the research study: (a) African American, woman, 40 years of age or older; (b) ability to communicate in English language effectively; (c) no previous or present diagnosis of breast cancer; (d) willingness to share their personal barriers, stereotype, status, culture, attitudes, beliefs, and how these factors could influence their breast cancer screening.

I e-mailed the participant a copy of the consent form, as well as confirmed the time and meeting place that had been arranged by the facility site. Once we were in a private interview room, I confirmed that there were no questions regarding the process and asked the participant to sign the consent form, provide me with her contact information if she wished to review the transcript of the interview, and/or wished to receive the results of the study. The participant wished to receive both and provided her contact information.

I started the recording and began asking the interview questions and making observation notes. Based upon the pilot participant's answers, I wrote down additional prompts and questions that were triggered by her responses. The interview lasted approximately 48 minutes. In closing, I thanked the participant for her cooperation and confirmed that I would e-mail the transcript for approval within 5 days (see Interview Protocol in Appendix B).

The pilot study went well. There were no technical problems with the recording equipment, and all the paperwork was in order. I gained more insight into my study through the pilot interview. Scheduling a time with the volunteer for the pilot interview was comparatively easier than with some of the actual participants. I found the practice of using the recording device and asking the questions improved my confidence in proceeding with the actual study. No changes were made to planned procedures as a consequence of my pilot study.

Setting

The 14 interviews were conducted in a private room located on the premises of the participants' church in an urban east coast region. Permission to use this setting was granted per the letter of cooperation agreement. The advantage of using this location was to make it as convenient and time efficient as possible for the participants. During the interview, I encountered some challenges. There were disturbances from the shouting of some children playing on a nearby playground. A participant had to leave for about 20 minutes because she needed to ensure that the sandwiches she and her group prepared for a shelter home for some homeless people would get delivered to them on time. This required me to pause the recording. Another participant was interrupted by a church member who had a question.

Demographics

The study participants consisted of 14 African American women. The age of the participants ranged from 40 years to 62 years with an average age of 50.07 years. All participants considered themselves African American with the ability to communicate effectively in English language. Eleven of the participants were either working or had worked in the health care sector. One of the participants was a teacher. One participant worked as a guard. Another participant worked as a nanny. Ten of the participants stated that they belonged to the middle class while four stated they were poor.

Data Collection

Data were collected from 14 African American women via one-on-one interviews. Each participant was asked 21 questions [See Interview Protocol in Appendix B] regarding her perceptions on different things regarding breast cancer screening and prevention. I interviewed all the participants and was the one who asked all the questions. The presentation of the interview questions to each participant was similar. However, variations occurred in the follow up questions and prompts depending on the response given by the participant. The interviews lasted for between 15-45 minutes. All the participants provided appropriate body language and eye contact, used a friendly tone in their voice, and they appeared very interested in the topic. Observation guide notes maintained during the interview provided a secondary data source (Appendix H) Variations were observed in regard to the thought and detail put into each of the responses by different participants.

All interviews were audio-taped and later transcribed. The transcriptions were reviewed to identify the obvious themes. The themes were coded, and their subcategories identified. The NVivo10 software was used to compare the themes that were identified.

Data Analysis

Interpretative phenomenological analysis was used to try to understand each participant's personal and social world. Six steps of data analysis were adopted according to the Smith, Jarman, and Osborn (1999) six–step analytical process: (a) looking for themes; (b) looking for connection; (c) producing a table of themes; (d) continuing the analysis with other cases; (e) creating a master list of themes and (f) writing up the findings.

The fourteen interviews were completed, and data saturation was achieved. By the time of interviewing participant 12 and 13, I realized that the information I was receiving was just a repetition of what I had received from earlier interviews. At this point, I realized that I had reached data saturation. Interviewing participant 14 was just to make sure that no new themes emerged, which later confirmed data saturation. Saturation occurred when all 21 questions were totally explored in detail and no new themes gained from additional interviews. I imported the recordings to NVivo10 and transcribed appropriately. I highlighted the questions following the research questions that they aimed to address. I did a systematic review of each transcript as relating to the research questions they addressed. I, then, extracted and compiled the key ideas and phrases from each transcript and the complied data was reviewed to identify themes. Each of the identified themes was assessed with an aim of determining the relationship they had with the category relating to a research question. Subthemes supporting the themes were identified from the rest of the data and noted accordingly.

I reviewed the transcripts again and noted any new themes as they emerged. Connections between the new and the old themes were then assessed in order to come up with a master list of themes. Once themes, subthemes, and new themes were noted and connections made, the transcripts were reviewed again to find and highlight quotes that were in support of the themes and the subthemes. Unconnected information to other themes was set aside if the information could not be established by data in the transcripts.

After gathering all the themes, the significance of the text supporting the themes determined whether a theme was listed on the master list of themes. I assessed this significance through word frequency, text search query, and coding query in NVivo10. NVivo10 also aided in storing and organizing data for easier, faster, and more accurate way of assessing the significance of the text supporting themes. The master list was used to create the report of the participants' responses during the interview. The master list of themes also aimed to cover the research questions.

Evidence of Credibility, Transferability, Dependability, and Confirmability

The research design and methods described in Chapter 3 were followed throughout the data collection and data analysis process. The participants that met the inclusion criteria and signed the consent form were the only ones allowed to participate in interviews. A question in the interview process also ascertained that the women met the inclusion criteria. Throughout the interviews, I used consistent questioning methods. To avoid researcher bias, I used the bracketing technique by writing memos throughout data collection as a means of evaluating and reflecting upon my engagement with the data. I maintained transferability by ensuring that I described and precisely documented the study participants' perspective and the statements central to the research. To establish dependability, I used audit trails and triangulation. My information resources included participants experiences gathered through interviews, and documented information. As a second source of information, I took observation notes and compared them with the responses from the participants. To enhance confirmability, I ensured to interpret and conclude research finding solely from data collected. I was mindful to observe rather than dictate the direction of the interviews and asked the study participants for clarification of any unfamiliar words.

Results

Table 2. Knowledge on breast cancer screening

Theme	Subthemes
Knowledge of Breast Cancer Screening	Participants showed understanding of the recommendations on mammogram and self-examination recommendations. All participants mentioned and correctly described the mammogram and self-breast examination procedures. (P1-P14). All the participants had some knowledge on mammogram and self-breast examination. Findings indicate that knowledge of recommendations on breast cancer screening may not be a major issue affecting utilization of breast cancer screening resources among African American women.
	Knowledge of breast cancer screening and recommendations has minimal effect on utilization of breast cancer screening and resources. (P1-P14). Despite the knowledge on breast cancer screening, five participants (P1, P4, P6, P7, and P11) did not utilize the available

	resources showing that knowledge has minimal effect on utilization of resources.
	Findings indicate that creating awareness may need to shift from focusing too much on the recommendations
Need for more education among African American women. (P1-P14).	All participants emphasized on the need for more education among African American women.
	The findings indicated a need for continued education among African American women on breast cancer screening.

When answering the question of their understanding of breast cancer screening and prevention, all participants mentioned mammogram and self-breast examination. Every participant at least had some knowledge of mammogram and self-breast examination as screening and preventive measures (P1-P14). Even the participants who said they did not do mammogram screening and they did not intend to do them, said they would encourage other African American women to go for screening; thus, they understood the benefits of breast cancer screening. Participants 1 and 4 statements demonstrate this clearly.

When asked how her concerns about participating in breast cancer screening and her awareness level about breast cancer screening affect her utilization of the available screening resources, participant 1(P1) said that she believes that "it (breast cancer screening) is not healthy," and she has a knowledge of natural health care that allows her to make preferences against breast cancer screening. On the other hand, on the advice to African American women, P1 encouraged them to be "proactive and take available screening resources," although she has her preferences against them.

P4 said that she has good knowledge of the recommendations of breast cancer screening and prevention since she has been in the medical field for a long time. However, following the recommendations is the issue. On how her awareness level affects her participation in screening, participant 4 said that instead of mammogram, she does self examination. She said that she wouldn't go for mammogram because of fear of getting a positive result and that it was better if she does not know. On the other hand, participant 4 encouraged African American women to go for screening despite saying that she would not participate in it. On the question of her advice to African American women, participant 4's advice was that she encourages them to go for screening and by all means have mammograms and do self-examination.

Table 3. Knowledge of available resources

Theme	Subthemes
Knowledge of available resources	Limited knowledge on free breast cancer screening resources (P1-P14). All the participants did not show substantive knowledge on the available breast cancer screening resources. Findings indicate a need to educate African American women on the available breast cancer screening resources in their community.
	Inadequate knowledge of procedures to get available resources limits utilization (P1-P14) All participants did not show substantive knowledge on how to access available resources in their community.

The finding indicates a need to focus on educating people on the procedures to access available breast cancer screening resources in their communities.

It is evident that most participants knew about the recommendations about breast cancer screening, demonstrated by the responses to the question about the same during the interview (P1-P14). Only one participant, that is participant 11, said that she did not know about the recommendation on mammogram. Even so, she had heard about mammograms and knew that she should do it, which was demonstrated by her response to the question on what she understood by breast cancer screening and responses to the question on the resources available in her community. On her understanding of breast cancer screening, she said that it was by checking her breasts herself or through mammogram. On the question of the available resources in their community, she said that she knew a little from her daughter who talks about it and her daughter told her about mammogram and had been encouraging her to do it, but she refused it and laughed at her daughter. This demonstrates that even participant 11 had some knowledge on the recommendations about mammogram screening. Despite this knowledge, some of the African American women did not go for screening as recommended (P1, P4, P6,

P7, P11), due to various reasons. Statements from participant 4 and participant 7 will demonstrate this.

Participant 4 said that she had good knowledge of the recommendations since she has been working in the medical field for a long time. However, following the recommendations was the issue. Participant 7 said she knew about the recommendations about going for a mammogram after the age of 40 years. She said that at her age she should have gone for the mammogram, and it was not because of lack of knowledge about the recommendations but because of her fears.

It is evident that there is need for more education about breast cancer screening among African American women. Many participants said that more education was needed to increase awareness of the same (P1, P2, P6, P7, P9, P12). Statements from participant 2 and participant 12 demonstrate the need for more education about breast cancer screening among African American women. The participants stressed the importance of education among African American women. The statements below demonstrate this clearly.

On the belief and attitude towards breast cancer screening, participant 2 said that breast cancer screening has helped women identify breast cancer at an early stage. She adds that screening should be encouraged, and awareness introduced through continued education. On the advice for health care providers, participant 2 said "sometimes when people have a problem with their breasts most of the times it is because they did not know....education, information, creating awareness is what healthcare providers should do." On the advice for health care providers, participant 12 encouraged the health care providers to offer free mammogram days for anybody to come in and participate and provide more education about examination and screening.

This study showed that African American women lack information on the available resource for breast cancer screening and prevention and how to get access to the resources. Most of the participants were not sure about the availability of free breast cancer screening resources in their community. Some participants admitted to not knowing of the available resources in their communities and the procedure of getting the available resources. Only participant 9 described the procedure of accessing free mammogram screening although most of them indicated that they thought it was there. The following statements from various participants demonstrate that there is general lack of information on the available resources and the process of accessing them.

Participant 1 said that she did not think that she would be correct in the procedure of assessing available resources. However, when answering the question on the available resources in her community, she said that there are free mammograms in some clinics for people and it is displayed that hospitals have free mammograms.

When answering the question on the available resources in her community, Participant 11 said that she did not really know about them. Her daughter told her about mammograms, but she did not want anybody to see or touch her breasts. She confirmed that she did not know about the seriousness of the procedure. From this statement, it shows that she did not bother to ask or find out the available resources since she was uninterested.

When answering the question on the available resources and the procedure to access the available resources in her community, Participant 6 demonstrated that she was very knowledgeable about them. She said that the available resources are the library, public health facilities, all health care providers, TV, Radio, and Facebook. When asked about the procedure to access available resources, Participant 6 demonstrated that she did not know the procedure of accessing the available resources in her community. She said that the process starts from the gynecologist and her. She added that what she is doing is to educate and watch her diet.

Table 4. Genetic stereotypes regarding the utilization of resources

Stereotype that genetics dictate affect utilization of breast cancer screening resources (P1, P2, P8, P9, P14)	Those with family history of breast cancer think they can do nothing about it (P1, P2). P1 and P2 emphasized on the behavior of African American women to ignore screening on the belief that family history of breast cancer predisposes that person to breast cancer and death.

The stereotype discourages African American women from utilizing breast cancer screening resources, thus a barrier.

Those with no family history of breast cancer think they cannot get it (P8, P9, P14)

P8, P9 and P14 emphasized on the behavior of African American women to ignore breast cancer screening recommendations on the belief that they are safe because their families have no history of breast cancer.

This stereotype that a person is safe because she does not come from a family with a history of breast cancer prevents people from following breast cancer screening recommendations and thus a barrier.

Five of the participants indicated that there is a belief among African American women that breast cancer is hereditary (P1, P2, P8, P9, P14). The stereotype affects screening behaviors and attitudes in a way that a woman who comes from a family with a history of breast cancer will tend to think that she cannot do anything about it and that she will probably get it and die (P1, P2). The statements below by Participants 1 and 2 demonstrate this tendency.

Participant 1

Breast cancer might be genetic, but lifestyle pulls the gun. Stereotypes play a role because some think it is genetic and think they can do nothing about it.

Participant 2

The understanding of breast cancer prevention and screening is that education and awareness are the most important thing. Other options to consider are self-breast examination, monthly routine self-breast examination, going to the doctor and radiology. Everybody can be involved no matter the genetics. Advice to African American women is that health is wealth, and it is a privilege which they can create and help put into place; they have a duty to humanity to live their part. They should not think that "my family had breast cancer, my aunt had breast cancer, my mother had breast cancer, my aunt on my father's side had breast cancer and they died from it and so they can do nothing. But they can change their DNA by doing what they did not do right."

Women from families without breast cancer history will think that they are safe and that they cannot get breast cancer. They, therefore, tend to think that it is not necessary for them to participate in screening. This may be facilitated by the fact that the recommendation for screening is emphasized to women who come from families with a history of breast cancer. While it is true that such women have increased risk of acquiring breast cancer than others, it sends the wrong signals to African American women who interpret it that if they come from a family with a history of breast cancer, they will get it and die, and they cannot do anything about it. And those whose families have no history of the same think they are safe. Statements from P8, P9, and P14 demonstrate this stereotype and its effect on breast cancer screening behaviors.

Participant 8

One of her personal barriers is that she believes that "if you are a healthy person, eat well, and have no other disease and no family history of breast cancer you will be fine"

Participant 9

People should screen no matter the family history and age. Do self examination usually after the monthly period or date of your birthday, if you are menopausal.

Participant 14

There is a tendency of thinking that it is hereditary and hence they do not go for screening because they think they are safe. Do screening regularly. Some women don't do self-examination as frequently as required. Take it seriously.

Table 5. Cancer screening and cultural beliefs

Conflict with Cultural Beliefs	Some aspects of screening are against the cultural beliefs of African Americans thus hindering utilization of breast screening resources (P1, P3, P5, P11, P12) Touching own breasts, an aspect associated with self-breast examination conflicts with the culture of the African Americans. This may be a barrier to utilization of available breast cancer screening resources. Letting another person, other than a person's husband touch a woman's breasts, an aspect associated with mammogram breast cancer screening was against the cultural beliefs of some participants. This may be a barrier to utilization of breast cancer screening resources. The findings indicate that the features that conflict with African American cultural beliefs may play

94

part as a barrier to breast cancer screening among African American women.

An aspect of breast cancer screening procedure may also limit the participation of African American women in breast cancer screening. Breast cancer screening involves another person touching and lifting a woman's breasts. In the case of self-examination, the procedure involves the woman touching to feel lumps in her own breasts.

Five of the participants expressed the touching and handling of breasts as a concern, which many referred to as "playing with the breasts." (P1, P5, P11, P12). They suggested that when it comes to mammogram, it would have been better if they were allowed to handle their own breasts through instruction from the technician. Two of the participants (P2, P3) said that touching their own breasts was also a challenge. This is a cultural belief as they think it is not normal for them to do so (P1, P2, P3, P5, P11, P12. The statements below from some of the participants will demonstrate these beliefs.

Participant 2

Participant 2 expressed concerns about the self-examination method. She said that "Initially to be fiddling with myself and massaging my own breasts didn't really make sense to me".

Participant 5

When asked about the most challenging aspect when she participated in breast cancer screening, P5 said that she was hesitant about showing her breasts as it was not modest. Her concern was about being bare, the breasts being exposed. However, she got over it after several screenings.

Participant 12

When asked about the type of screening she had undergone though, Participant 12 said that she has had self examination and mammogram. She said that "the pressing is so hard,

touching and playing with your breasts, it's okay but I would prefer somebody not touching or playing with my breasts."

Table 6. Normal behavior regarding screening

The Norm	It is normal for people not to go for any check-up among African Americans (P1, P2, P10, P11, and P12). P1, P2, P10, P11, and P12 emphasized the effect of the norm of African Americans not going for check-ups. They feel they are healthy, believe that is God is in control, or think that they would look weak if they went for check-ups. This norm is continued when it comes to breast cancer screening. The norm of not going for check-ups is therefore, a barrier to breast

cancer screening among African American women.

Culture also affects participation in breast cancer screening in that it is a normal thing among African American people not to go for medical checkup. This is evident as many of the participants said that many African American people do not take their health seriously (P1, P2, P10, P11, P12) or thought that they were healthy people. Some of the participants, P7 and P11, also admitted to not taking their health seriously, which was a hindrance to participation in breast cancer screening. The following statements from some of the participants demonstrate the aspect that it is a cultural thing not to go for any medical checkup, unless when they are ill.

Participant 1

Women don't feel like going to hospital because they feel it is not necessary unless they become very ill. Preventive measures are not part of the culture.

Participant 2

African American women feel that it is not necessary to go for screening, but with education it can improve.

Participant 10

Some of the friends and people she interacts with think it is not important. Some of them do not have health care insurance. Africans are not taught to do it culturally.

Participant 12

Africans don't believe in health care much. They believe they are okay as long as they are well. They think that they do not need it.

Other factors affecting breast cancer screening behaviors among African American women

Table 7. Other factors affecting screening in African American Women

Procedure of Screening	The mammogram procedure is painful and physical discomfort during screening may affect utilization of screening (P1, P4-P8, P10-P13)
	The discomfort discourages people from participating and thus a barrier to breast cancer screening.
	Coldness of breast cancer screening machines may affect utilization of breast cancer screening.

P9, P10 and P12 raised issues of the coldness of the machine, which shows is a potential hindrance to participating in breast cancer screening.

Apart from culture and stereotype and education, other factors that may affect breast cancer screening behaviors among African American women include the procedure of breast cancer screening (P1-P13) and fear of the unknown (P3, P4, P7, P10). On the procedure of breast cancer screening, 10 of the participants said that it was painful, and others said that the machines were too cold and hence uncomfortable.

Although some of the participants went for screening as recommended despite having these challenges, they would prefer it changed. Some of the participants said that it was the pain and the discomfort that hindered them from participating in breast cancer screening. The fact that these women did not participate because of the challenges means that the challenges would affect breast cancer screening behaviors among African American women.

Three participants raised issues of the coldness of the mammogram machine as a challenge when they did it, which made them uncomfortable. The participants thought that making the machines warmer would enhance their experience and/or participation in breast cancer screening (P9, P10, and P12). The statements of the participants below will explain the concerns raised about the coldness of the machine and the procedure of breast cancer screening in general.

Participant 9

People complain about breasts being pressed and the coldness of the machine.

Participant 10

The most challenging thing was waiting when they said they found something was scary was very scary. The experience called booby smashing, the cold. It doesn't bother me but I wish it was warmer. The factors that could enhance the experience and/or utilization of breast cancer screening resources would be warm equipment and nice personality.

Participant 12

The most challenging things were touching, pulling, and smashing that you are uncomfortable for some time and the temperatures are cold making the nipples be pointing. To enhance the experience the temperatures should not be very cold.

Ten of the participants expressed concerns about the mammogram screening being painful (P1, P4-P8, P10-P13). Some of the participants who did not go for breast cancer screening as recommended listed the painful mammogram experience as the hindrance (P4, P7). The following statements from some of the participants will illustrate the concerns.

Participant 1

Most challenging aspect about the screening was that it was very painful because of the pressing.

Participant 4

I don't like screening because it is painful.

Mammogram is extremely painful, and breasts easily bruise and very ticklish. She would not want to be touched by anyone else.

Have had a mammogram and she felt that she was being handled too much, there was pain, sores, and bruises.

Participant 7

The concerns about breast cancer screening are horror stories she has heard about mammogram. She has had no mammogram, but she does self examination. The burning sensation, a radiating pain going across chest, nipples sores and burning a little bit are things that have made her not participate in screening despite knowing its importance. However, she says that she will go for mammogram within the next week or two. She said that the breasts are large and sensitive, and she feared going for breast cancer screening because of the pain.

Table 8. Fear and breast cancer screening

Fear	Fear of the unknown may be affect utilization of screening resources (P3, P4, P7, and P10).
	Four of the participants indicated that fear that they might actually have cancer as a barrier to breast cancer screening among African women.

Fear of the unknown is yet another thing that could affect breast cancer screening behavior. Many participants raised concerns that they fear a positive result when they go for breast cancer screening, which limits their participation in the same (P3, 4, 7, 10).

Statements from some of the participants on the same that will explain this aspect are as follows:

Participant 3

The most challenging aspect about breast cancer screening is being afraid of what could happen.

Participant 4

I don't like screening because it is painful, and I am fearful of breast cancer detection. I do not do regular screening because of the fear. At 62 years old, I have only done it twice. Participant 4 says that instead of mammogram she does self examination and wouldn't go for mammogram because of fear of positive result and that its better she does not know.

Participant 10

The concern she has is fear that she may find out something she does not want to find out, for every woman there is one of those things you don't wanna find.

The most challenging aspect of breast cancer screening was waiting when they said they found something was scary was very scary.

Summary

Most of the participants showed substantial knowledge of breast cancer screening. All the participants had at least some knowledge of self-breast examination and mammogram as breast cancer screening methods. Additionally, most of the participants showed understanding of the benefits of breast cancer screening. Most of the people knew how to go about the self-breast examination to check for lumps. Additionally, most of them had gone for at least one session of mammogram and all of them had at least done self-breast examination. In addition, most of them knew about the recommendations on breast cancer screening as regular self-breast examination and yearly mammogram once a person is over 40. However, despite the knowledge on breast cancer screening and the recommendations about the same, some of them did not go for breast screening due to different reasons. However, most of them did self-breast examination as required. Most of the participants said that the awareness of the same among African American women was limited and suggested education as a way to increase the awareness.

The observation of the know-how about benefits and recommendation, which contrasted with the participation in breast cancer screening, suggests need for more education on accessing available resources and dispelling misleading myths and beliefs about breast cancer screening.

The participants expressed a general limited know-how of the available resources in their community and the procedure of accessing the resources. Although a few of them admitted to not knowing of the available resources and the procedure of accessing the resources, their answers to the questions regarding the same showed a general limited know-how especially on the procedure of accessing the available resources. Many of the participants were not sure of the free mammogram resources in their community and did not know the procedure of accessing the same. Some of the participants admitted to not knowing of the available resources. Culture and stereotype were found to be a noteworthy factor affecting participation in breast cancer screening among African American women. The stereotype that genetics dictate who gets breast cancer is a major factor affecting breast cancer screening behaviors.

There is a stereotype among African American women that people from families with no history of breast cancer are safe from breast cancer. Those with families with a history of breast cancer believe they are predisposed to get breast cancer and die, which makes them see breast cancer screening as unnecessary. On the issue of culture, handling of breasts by the screening technician or oneself is against the culture of African Americans thus affecting their breast cancer screening behaviors. Going for screening and exposing one's breasts and letting the technician touch them make them feel bare and indecent. The findings show that the norm for not going for medical checkups among African Americans is another cultural factor that affects breast screening behaviors. As one of the participants put it, "it is not in their culture to go for medical checkups. African Americans tend to think that so long as they do not feel sick, they are okay and do not need any checkup, including breast cancer screening…"

Other factors that may affect breast cancer screening behaviors are the procedure of the screening and fear of unknown. Most of the participants did not have pleasant experiences when they had gone for mammogram screening. The participants expressed concerns on the pain that the machine causes and the coldness of the machine. From their responses, it was evident that the mammogram procedure left them feeling very physically uncomfortable. Some participants listed this as a factor in why they did not go for screening. Fear of unknown also featured significantly in the responses to why African American women and was a factor that could affect breast cancer screening behaviors. Some participants feared that the results may come out positive after they have had breast cancer screening and thus feared the experience of having breast cancer and the treatment process. The participants said that they would prefer not knowing some things, and having breast cancer is one of those things. In Chapter 5, I offer detailed discussion, conclusions, and recommendations based upon the results of my study with` comparison to the literature review.

Chapter 5:

Discussion, Conclusions, and

Recommendations

Introduction

The primary purpose of this study was to explore individual barriers to breast cancer screening among African American women, 40 years and older, to better understand why breast cancer continues to be one of the principal sources of mortality among African American women. Purposes also included identifying barriers to preventive screening for breast cancer among African American women and to explore the influence of personal barriers, stereotypes, socioeconomic status, culture, attitudes, and beliefs on the behavior of African American women in regard to breast cancer screening. The chapter also presents (a) an analysis of findings based on the conceptual framework, (b) limitations of the study, (c) recommendations, (d) implications for positive change, and (e) conclusions. For this phenomenological study, in-depth interviews were conducted with 14 African American women in an urban East Coast city.

The barriers to breast cancer screening among African American women were as follows: limited information, stereotypic beliefs, influence of the culture, the screening procedure, and fear of the unknown. Socioeconomic status was not seen as a significant factor that affects breast cancer screening behaviors.

According to Smith and Osborn (2003), the use of phenomenological design can make it easier to understand participants' personal and social world, particularly how participants make sense of their world. A gap exists in understanding the barriers to breast cancer screening among African American women who are 40 years and older.

Attaining the views of African American women who are over 40 years old can inform researchers of what African American women think needs to be done to increase participation in breast cancer screening among African American women who are 40 years and older.

In this chapter, the results will be interpreted. In addition, an explanation of the agreement with, disagreement with, or an extension of the understanding of previous research on barriers to breast cancer screening among African American women will be presented.

Interpretation of the Findings

I collected and analyzed the data for this qualitative, phenomenological study using the steps recommended by Smith, Jarman, and Osborn (1999). In addition to hand coding, I analyzed the transcriptions in NVivo10 software for content and word analysis which helped in data triangulation and results to have a high level of trustworthiness and credibility. The major themes of the study were evaluated alongside the literature review. I offer interpretations of how these findings integrate into the field of barriers to breast cancer screening.

Results, Confirmation, Disconfirmation, or Extension of Knowledge

Knowledge on breast cancer screening recommendations was found to be substantial among African American women. All the participants demonstrated knowledge of the recommendation for yearly mammogram exam. However, there was limited knowledge on the available resources in the community for breast cancer screening and how to access the resources. Participants expressed a need for more education to African American women on breast cancer screening. Therefore, education focusing on the available resources and how to access available resources is a way to increase awareness of breast cancer screening among African American women. Stereotypes and culture were found to have an effect on the utilization of breast cancer screening resources. The stereotype that genetics dictate who gets and who dies from breast cancer is a factor that affects utilization of breast cancer screening resources.

The culture of the norm of people attending medical checkups is a cultural aspect that influences utilization of the resources too. Some aspects of breast cancer screening like letting another person touch a woman's breasts conflicts with cultural beliefs and limits utilization of the breast cancer screening resources. Other factors that may affect utilization of breast cancer screening resources are the pain associated with the procedure, the coldness of the machines, and the fear of the unknown.

Health care utilization is influenced by need-related factors, supply-induced factors, and social characteristics among others. The behavioral model of health services use (BMHSU) is a model incorporating individual and contextual determinants of utilization of health services (Andersen, 1995). According to the model, the major components of contextual determinants are the predisposing factors, enabling factors, and need factors. Predisposing factors are factors that incline people to use or not use healthcare and may include political perspectives, cultural norms, and collective and organizational values. Enabling factors are organizational and financing factors that enable health services to be utilized. Enabling factors may include health policies, resources available within the community, health insurance status, and income among others. Need factors include perceived need, evaluated need, population need and environmental need for health services. The findings of the study confirmed the above model.

The effect of stereotypes and culture, limited knowledge on the resources and the procedure to access available breast cancer screening resources are predisposing factors as explained by the behavioral model of health services use model. These factors align African American women to not using breast cancer screening resources. The pain, the coldness of the machines, and the fear of the unknown are the enabling factors that influence utilization of breast cancer screening resources. These factors make breast cancer screening less desirable and thus limit utilization of the same. Need factors include the perceived health among African American women who do not find any need for health care, which prevents them from utilizing the available breast cancer screening resources.

Rice (2000) hypothesized that any health-related action would depend on two factors: a) Existence of sufficient motivation or a health concern, which would make the salient health issues relevant; b) the belief that someone is vulnerable to serious health condition of the perceived threat. The theory is known as the behavioral model of health services use. A belief exists that following health recommendations is beneficial in reducing the health threat, which is subjective to acceptable costs. The costs are the perceived barriers that a person must overcome to follow the health recommendations. According to Rice, behavioral change would need perceived seriousness of the disease, perceived increased likelihood of developing the disease, and perceived benefits of following the recommendations must outweigh the cost of overcoming the perceived barriers. The findings of this study confirm this hypothesis.

All the five participants (P1, P4, P6, P7, and P11), who did not follow the breast cancer screening, fell in one or more of the reasons not to follow recommendations. Although other participants had perceived barriers, they had a high perceived risk and seriousness of breast cancer, and the benefits of breast cancer screening outweighed the perceived barriers.

Participant 1 did not follow recommendations because of her belief in natural health, which means that her perception of the likelihood of developing breast cancer is minimized, although she has a perceived seriousness of breast cancer. Participant 4 did not follow recommendations because she never wants to know the outcome and she thought she was being handled too much. In this case, the participant recognized the seriousness of the disease and the high likelihood of her getting it. However, the barriers, which are knowing and the discomfort in the screening process outweighs the perceived benefits. The participant found no benefits of breast cancer screening as she thought that it would just cause more trouble. Participant 6 did not follow breast cancer screening recommendations because of the financial issues. In this case, the participant does recognize the seriousness and the likelihood of developing breast cancer, and she has perceived benefits of breast cancer screening. However, the barrier, which in this case is finances. outweighs the perceived benefits. Participant 7 did not follow the breast cancer screening recommendations because she feared the process of screening. However, she knows the benefits and has high perceived risk and seriousness. However, the cost of

breast cancer screening outweighs the benefits. Participant 11 did not follow recommendations because of lack of knowledge about it and the free services available. This means that the perceived barriers outweigh the benefits since she does not have any perceived benefits towards the same.

Philips et al. (2001) found out that themes between middle-income and low-income African American women on breast cancer screening were similar. However, there existed differences in the types of barriers among these women. While low-income earners expressed accessibility of healthcare as barrier to not participate in screening. Middle-income women had other barriers. This study has replicated these findings. This study did not find socioeconomic status as a significant barrier to breast cancer screening among African American women since although most participants thought that their socioeconomic status influenced their screening behaviors, only one participant indicated that socioeconomic status is the reason she does not participate in breast cancer screening. However, this study was limited since most of the women interviewed belonged to the same socioeconomic status. Further investigation would be needed to find out whether socioeconomic status had any effect on breast cancer screening behaviors.

Ahmed et al (2004) set out a study of the barriers and facilitating factors among regularly compliant and underserved women, of which African American women were a part. My study found out those healthcare system barriers as one of the many barriers to breast cancer screening. Pain and the discomfort of the mammography machine were part of the barriers found out by this study. This is confirmed by my research study that found out that the procedure of breast cancer screening could affect breast cancer screening behaviors. Mooradian (2010) also found out that pain and embarrassment that is associated with mammogram screening was a barrier to participating in breast cancer screening among minority group of women. In the current study, embarrassment has been linked to culture.

Ogedegbe et al. (2005) found out that among minority women in America, including African American women and Latino women, patient attitudes and beliefs, accessibility of services, and social network experiences were barriers to cancer screening. According to the research, lack of knowledge about cancer screening, fear of cancer and pain were part of the attitudes and beliefs. My study confirms these barriers specifically on breast cancer screening as fear, pain, and insufficient knowledge especially about the available screening resources and the procedure to access them were significant barriers to breast cancer screening. The study by Ogedegbe and colleagues also found out that the perception that people do not need the test was a significant barrier to breast cancer screening. This was in line with the current study. My research findings are that the perception of not needing the test was as an influence of culture and stereotypes among African American women.

Bastien (2005) found out that African American women have knowledge about breast cancer screening and know about the recommendations. This is confirmed by my study that found out that African American women had adequate knowledge on breast cancer screening and recommendations about the same. However, the finding of my study contrasts Lukwago et al.'s (2003) study which had reported lack of knowledge on recommendations and need for breast cancer screening.

My study also found stereotypes to be factors affecting breast cancer screening behaviors–specifically the stereotype that genetics dictate who gets breast cancer and who does not. In this regard, those who think that they have the genes of getting breast cancer, feel that there is nothing they can do to stop that. Those who feel that they do not have the genes of getting breast cancer; they see themselves as safe and hence do not see the need for healthcare. This phenomenon can be explained by the hypothesis that health- related action depends on the existence of sufficient motivation or a health concern, and the belief of vulnerability to a serious health condition. However, perceived benefits must be greater than the perceived costs. In either group, one condition works against the other. There are those who think that they are predisposed to breast cancer and dying from it, and the benefits of breast cancer screening fail to outweigh the costs of taking a health-related action, in this case breast cancer screening. This group does not find any benefit in breast cancer screening since they think that even if they went for screening, they would still get breast cancer and die from it. Participant 2 demonstrated the reasoning of this group very well when she said that she thinks that because her mother and their two aunts died from breast cancer, she will also get it and die from it irrespective of the preventive actions she takes. Whereas this group of women has a high perceived risk and high perceived seriousness of the disease, the group does not participate in breast screening because the women think that it would not be helpful. Therefore, they would not be willing to overcome the barriers of participating in breast cancer screening. The group that thinks that they do not have the genes of getting breast cancer, and thus feel safe, do not perceive high risk of contracting the disease. Although they perceive seriousness of the disease, the fact that they do not perceive themselves as likely to get the disease makes them reluctant to participate in breast cancer screening.

Brandon and Proctor (2010) found out that African Americans health perceptions are often inconsistent with their actual health. These perceptions about their health then influence the value they place in health behaviors. My study found that one of the barriers to participation in breast cancer screening among African American women was that it was the norm of the society not to go for any health checkups unless they are very ill. This can be explained by the Brandon and Proctor finding that health perceptions about themselves affect the breast cancer screening behaviors. African American women think that their health is okay, that they live healthy lifestyles, and that God is in control and as long as they are not in pain or feeling sick, they are healthy. Due to these perceptions among African American women, they would not go for the screening. I found from my in-depth studies that this behavior is a cultural aspect since it is the norm of that particular society.

Contribution to Science

This study uses the phenomenological approach, which demonstrates the importance of lived experience. The study seeks personal perceptions and experiences of African American women that give important insight on the beliefs, attitudes, and perceived barriers to breast cancer screening among themselves as African American women. Perceived barriers should be considered when developing intervention measures to ensure heightened awareness about breast cancer screening among African Americans. This is to ensure complete understanding of the situation at hand and come up with workable solutions.

This research also contributes to science by further supporting behavioral model of health services use as a practical model for evaluating the factors influencing utilization of health care resources. The research also supports the behavioral model of health services use as a practical theory in the field of perceived barriers to taking health- related actions. The study results show that the theory would affect behaviors regarding health-related actions such as breast cancer screening.

Contribution to Field

Barriers to breast cancer screening have consequences that result in deaths of many American citizens from breast cancer. Breast cancer continues to be one of the principle causes of death in women in African American societies. When compared to other societies, African American women are likely to die from breast cancer than other groups in America. Many national, state, and community programs such as National Breast and Cervical Cancer Early Detection Program (NBCCEDP), Friend to Friend, Proactive System to Improve Breast Cancer Screening, and Mammography Promotion and Facilitated Appointments Through Community-based Influenza Clinics, (CDC, 2015; RTIPS, 2015) aim to increase awareness about breast cancer screening. Since African American women mortality rates are highest as a result of breast cancer, research investigating their perceptions is important.

I gathered detailed information on the perceptions of African American women regarding barriers to participating in breast cancer screening. These comprised of the participant's perceptions, knowledge, and experiences as regards breast cancer screening and the advice to African American women and health care providers as regards breast cancer screening. Further research on the perceived barriers to breast cancer screening can build upon my study's input. My study provides the planners of breast cancer screening intervention programs with important insight on awareness and effect of culture and stereotypes and the direction that they can follow to formulate their programs in such a way as to provide effective solutions and reduce breast cancer mortality among African American women.

Limitations

The study's participants were African American women from a church in an urban east coast region. Therefore, a limitation of the study would be that the findings represent a small non-probable sample that lives in a localized region and having similar socioeconomic status. The sample could also have been subjected to the awareness from the church and thus some of the perceptions and behaviors may fail to capture the general population's perceptions and behaviors. Generalizability cannot extend beyond this particular study sample. However, the in-depth interview approach provided insight and themes possibly applicable to similar type groups in the United States and other regions of the world. The completeness of understanding may also have been limited by the participants' limited amount of time. The interviews required 45-60 minutes of interview protocol for reflective answers. Some of the participants could only afford 15 minutes, which would be too short to conduct all the interview protocol. Most of the participants were busy people and scheduling interviews was a bit challenging. Additionally, there were interruptions in some of the interviews. Participants may have had inadequate time to elaborate their responses in order to save time. However, 14 in-depth interviews yielded saturation of data and allowed answering RQs. Insightful findings unique to this study that add to the literature were the following recommendations.

Recommendations

My study and a previous researcher (Bastien, 2005) have found that African American women are knowledgeable as regards the benefits of breast cancer screening and recommendations. However, African American women showed limited knowledge of the available resources in their community and the procedure of accessing the available resources. Additionally, participants indicated the need for continued education specifically addressing myths with regards to beliefs in genetics and destiny for no cures and awareness of breast cancer screening. Therefore, awareness programs should focus on educating African American women on the available resources in the community and how they can access them. Seminars and organizing health festivals could be a good way of educating the women in the societies. Aligning with church groups and other community groups among Africa American women would also help increase the awareness on available screening resources and how to access them easily. Additional investigation might be performed to illustrate the educational methods that would be most appropriate among African American women. My research has showed that stereotype and cultural influences are barriers to participating breast cancer screening. The findings have also been showed by other researchers (Brandon & Proctor, 2010; Ogededgbe et al., 2005). Therefore, planners of the awareness programs should consider the cultural aspects that are barriers to breast cancer screening such as the stereotype regarding genetics, the norm of people not going for checkups, and embarrassment. When talking about breast cancer screening among African American women, special emphasis should be put on these factors to educate the need for screening, the risk they have of contracting the disease, and the seriousness of the disease. The education about these things will specifically enhance the BMHSU factors and thus triggering behavioral change towards taking up the health act that is recommended, in this case breast cancer screening.

The procedure of breast cancer screening, which was deemed painful, was found to be a major barrier to participation in the same by this study and previous studies (Ahmed et al, 2004; Mooradian, 2010). Educating health care providers on the best procedures to improve the experience of those participating in breast cancer screening would help.

Additionally, more education on the seriousness of the disease and the high risk of getting it among African American women should be encouraged to ensure that the perceive barriers such as pain and discomfort are seen as acceptable costs for getting the benefits of breast cancer screening. Additional investigation needs to be done on whether the expertise and skill of the technician performing the screening has any effect on that person's experience. This would help women choose technicians who will enhance their experience hence encouraging others to participate.

Implications for Positive Social Change

This study has showed the factors that should be considered to improve on the awareness of breast cancer and ensure a positive behavioral change in terms of participation in breast screening. Awareness programs must shift from teaching about recommendations and focus on teaching about available resources and how to access them. The programs must also deal with stereotypes and cultural behaviors and beliefs that hinder utilization of breast cancer screening resources available in the community. The findings of this study should raise awareness of program organizers to create content that will address the actual lack of information such as informing people of the available breast cancer screening resources and how to access them. This way, there will be observable behavioral change towards embracing breast screening among African American women.

Conclusion

Understanding the perceptions, knowledge, and experiences of African American women provided insights of the perceived barriers to breast cancer screening, ways to increase awareness, and the effect of stereotypes on belief and behaviors regarding breast cancer screening. The findings of this study demonstrated that perceived barriers to breast cancer screening are lack of information, belief that genetics dictates who gets breast cancer, embarrassment, norm of people not going for health checkups, procedure of breast cancer screening, and fear. Awareness of breast cancer screening and prevention can be promoted through education, holding health festivals, and collaborating with the church and other community groups. Stereotypes and cultural aspects such as belief that genetics determine who gets breast cancer, the embarrassment of someone handling a woman's breasts, and norm of not going to health checkups creates barriers that are not worth overcoming as compared to the perceived risk of getting breast cancer and the seriousness of breast cancer. Breast cancer screening among Africa American women will increase if only education that teaches against dominant and retrogressive cultural beliefs such as the role of genetics and destiny in breast cancer is increased.

References

Adams, S. A., Smith, E. R., Hardin, J., Das, I. P., Fulton, J., & Hebert, J. R. (2009). Racial differences in follow-up of abnormal mammography findings among economically disadvantaged women. *Cancer, 115*(24), 5788-5797. doi: 10.1002/cncr.24633

Ahmadian, M., & Samah, A. A. (2013). Application of health behavior theories to breast cancer screening among Asian women. *Asian Pacific Journal of Cancer Prevention, 14*(7), 4005-4013. doi: 10.7314/APJCP.2013.14.7.4005

Ahmed, N. U., Fort, J. G., Elzey, J. D. & Bailey, S. (2004). Empowering factors in repeat mammography: Insights from the stories of undeserved women. Journal of Ambulatory Care Manage, 27(4), 348-355.

Ahmed, N. U., Fort, J. G., Fair, A. M., Semenya, K., & Haber, G. (2009). Breast cancer knowledge and barriers to mammography in a low-income managed care population. *Journal of Cancer Education, 24*(4), 261-266. doi: 10.1080/08858190902973077

Ahmed, N. U., Winter, K., Albatineh, A. N., & Haber, G. (2012). Clustering very low-income, insured women's mammography screening barriers into potentially functional subgroups. *Womens Health Issues, 22*(3), e259-e266. doi: 10.1016/j.whi.2012.02.001

Ajzen, I., Brown, T. C., & Carvajal, F. (2004). Explaining the discrepancy between intentions and actions: The case of hypothetical bias in contingent valuation. *Personality Social Psychology Bulletin, 30,* 1108. doi: 10.1177/0146167204264079

Alberta Health Services. (2010). Health promotion and behavior change theory. Retrieved from http://www.screeningforlife.ca/resources/Health%20 Promotion%20Evidence/Health%20Promotion%20Evidence/He alth%20Promotion%20and%20Behaviour%20Change%20Theo ry.pdf

Alexandraki, I., & Mooradian, A. D. (2010). Barriers related to mammography use of breast cancer screening among minority women. *Journal of the National Medical Association,102*(3), 2016-218. pmid:20355350

American Association of Cancer Research. (2011, March 1). Obesity may increase risk of triple-negative breast cancer. Retrieved from http://www.aacr.org/home/public--media/aacr-in-the-news.aspx?d=2276

American Cancer Society, Cancer Action Network. (2009). Cancer disparities: A chart book. Retrieved from http://action.acscan.org/site/DocServer/cancer-disparities-chartbook.pdf?docID=15341

American Cancer Society. (2009). Cancer facts and figures 2009. Retrieved from http://www.cancer.org/research/cancerfactsstatistics/cancerfacts

figures2009/index

American Cancer Society. (2011). Cancer facts and figures 2011.

Retrieved from

http://www.cancer.org/acs/groups/content/@epidemiologysurve

ilance/documents/document/acspc-029771.pdf

American Cancer Society. (2013a). Breast cancer facts & figures 2013-

2014. Retrieved from

http://www.cancer.org/acs/groups/content/@research/document

s/document/acspc-042725.pdf

American Cancer Society. (2013b). Cancer facts & figures for African

Americans 2013-2014. Retrieved from

http://www.cancer.org/acs/groups/content/

@epidemiologysurveilance /documents/document/acspc-

036921.pdf

American Cancer Society. (2013c). Cancer prevention & early

detection facts & figures. Retrieved from

http://www.cancer.org/research/cancerfactsfigures

/cancerpreventionearlydetectionfactsfigures/cancer-prevention-

early-detection-facts-figures-2013

American Cancer Society. (2015). Types of breast cancers. Retrieved

from http://www.cancer.org/cancer/breastcancer/

detailedguide/breast-cancer-breast-cancer-types

Andersen R. M., & Davidson, P. L. (2001). Improving access to care in

America: individual and contextual indicators. In: Andersen

RM, Rice TH, Kominski EF, editors. Changing the U.S. health

care system: key issues in health services, policy, and management. San Francisco, CA: Jossey-Bass; 2001. pp. 3–30

Andersen, R. M. (1995). Revisiting the behavioral model and access to medical care: Does it matter? *Journal of Health and Social Behavior, 36*(1), 1-10. doi: 10.2307/2137284

Anderson, R. M. (2008). National health surveys and the behavioral model of health services. *Medical Care, 46*, 647-653. doi: 10.1097/MLR.0b013e31817a835d

Autier, P., Boniol, M., La Vecchia, C., Vatten, L., Gavin, A., Héry, C., & Heanue, M. (2010). Disparities in breast cancer mortality trends between 30 European countries: retrospective trend analysis of WHO mortality database. *British Medical Journal, 341*, c3620. doi: 10.1136/bmj.c3620

Babitsch, B., Gohl, D., & von Lengerke, T. (2012). Re-revisiting Andersen's Behavioral Model of Health Services Use: a systematic review of studies from 1998-2011. *GMS Psycho-Social-Medicine, 9*. doi:10.3205/psm000089

Bandura, A., & Adams, N. E. (1977). Analysis of self-efficacy theory of behavioral change. *Cognitive Therapy Research, 1*, 287-310. doi: 10.1007/BF01663995

Banning, M. (2011). Black women and breast health: A review of the literature. *European Journal of Oncology Nursing, 15*(1), 16-22. doi: 10.1016/j.ejon.2010.05.005

Barcellos-Hoff, M. H. (2012). Does microenvironment contribute to the etiology of estrogen receptor-negative breast cancer? *Clinical*

Cancer Research, 19(3), 541-548. doi: 10.1158/1078-0432.CCR-12-2241

Bastien, N. E. (2005). Perceived barriers to breast cancer screening: A comparison of African American and European American women. Scholar Commons, University of South Florida

Bates, B., and Harris, T., M. (2004). The Tuskegee Study of Untreated Syphilis and Public Perceptions of Biomedical Research: A Focus Group Study. Journal of the National Medical Association, 96(8), 1051-64. Retrieved from ProQuest Central. (Document ID: 672913581

Batina, N. G., Trentham-Dietz, A., Gangnon, R. E., Sprague, B. L., Rosenberg, M. A., Stout, N. K., Alagoz, O. (2013). Variation in tumor natural history contributes to racial disparities in breast cancer stage at diagnosis. *Breast Cancer Research and Treatment, 138*(2), 519-528. doi: 10.1007/s10549-013-2435-z

Beatson, G. T. (1896). On the treatment of inoperable cases of carcinoma of the mamma: Suggestions for a new method of treatment, with illustrative cases. *The Lancet, 148*, b104-b107. doi: 10.1016/S0140-6736(01)72307-0

Black Women's Health Imperative. (n.d.). Black women and breast cancer: Surviving breast cancer through early detection and diagnosis. Retrieved from http://www.blackwomenshealth.org/issues-and-resources/black-women-and-breast-cancer/

Bowen, S. A., Williams, E. M., Stoneberg-Cooper, C. M., Glover, S. H., Williams, M. S., & Byrd, M. D. (2013). Effects of social injustice on breast health–seeking behaviors of low-income women. *American Journal of Health Promotion, 27*(4), 222-230. doi: 10.4278/ajhp.110505-QUAL-189

Boyle, P. (2012). Triple-negative breast cancer: Epidemiological considerations and recommendations. *Annals of Oncology, 23*(suppl. 6), vi7-vi12. doi: 10.1093/annonc/mds187

Brandon. J. L., & Proctor, L. (2010). Comparison of Health Perceptions and Health Status in African Americans and Caucasians. *Journal of National Medical Association, 102*(7):590-597.

Breast Care Site. (2009, September 7). African-Americans - cutting through culture. Retrieved from http://www.thebreastcaresite.com/after-surgery/african-americans-cutting-culture/

BreastCancer.org. (2011, November 30). No link between family history and risk for younger women. Retrieved from http://www.breastcancer.org/research-news/20111130

Breen, N., Gentleman, J. F., & Schiller, J. S. (2011). Update on mammography trends: Comparison of rates in 2000, 2005 and 2008. *Cancer, 117*(10), 2209-2218. doi: dx.doi.org/10.1002/cncr.25679

Cancer Research UK. (2010). Breast cancer incidence statistics. Retrieved from http://www.cancerresearchuk.org/cancer-

info/cancerstats/types/breast/incidence/uk-breast-cancer-
incidence-statistics

Cancer Research UK. (2013). Breast cancer genes. Retrieved from
http://www.cancerresearchuk.org/cancer-help/type/breast-
cancer/about/risks/breast-cancer-genes

Cardarelli, K. M., Ottenbacher, A., Linnear, K., Paul, M., Martin, M.,
Akinboro, O., Dallas Cancer Disparities Coalition Community
Advisory Board. (2013). Reducing breast cancer screening
barriers among underserved women in South Dallas. *TPHA
Journal, 65*(1), 14-91.

Centers for Disease Control and Prevention (2015).National Breast and
Cervical Cancer Early Detection Program
(NBCCEDP).http://www.cdc.gov/cancer/nbccedp/

Chatterjee, N., He, Y., & Keating, N. (2013). Racial differences in
breast cancer stage at diagnosis in the mammography era.
American Journal of Public Health, 103(1), 170-176. doi:
10.2105/AJPH.2011.300550

Cohen, S. S., Palmieri, R. T., Nyante, S. J., Korlek, D. O., Kim, S.,
Bradshaw, P., & Olshan, A. F. (2008). Obesity and screening
for breast, cervical, and colorectal cancer in women: A review.
Cancer, 112, 1892–1904. doi: 10.1002/cncr.23408

Collingridge, D., & Grant, E. (2008). The quality of qualitative
research. *American Journal of Medical Quality, 23*(5), 389-395.
doi: 10.1177/1062860608320646

Conway-Phillips, R., & Janusek, L. (2014). Influence of sense of coherence, spirituality, social support and health perception on breast cancer screening motivation and behaviors in African American Women. *ABNF Journal, 25*(3), 72-79.

Conway-Phillips, R., & Millon-Underwood, S. (2009). Breast cancer screening behaviors of African American women: A comprehensive review, analysis, and critique of nursing research. *The ABNF Journal, 20*(4), 97–101. Pmid: 19927894

Cooper, H. M. (1984). *The integrative research review: A systematic approach. Applied social research methods series* (Vol. 2). Beverly Hills, CA: Sage

Creswell, J. (2007). Qualitative Inquiry and Research Design: Choosing Among Five Approaches (2nd dd.). Thousand Oaks: Sage Publications.

Creswell, J. (2009). Research design. Qualitative, quantitative, and mixed methods approach. Los Angeles, CA. Sage Publications

Crosby, R.A, DiClemente, R.J., & Salazar, L.F. (2006). Research methods in health promotion. San Francisco, CA. Jossey-Bass.

Deavenport, A., Modeste, N., Marshak, H. H., & Neish, C. (2011). Closing the gap in mammogram screening: An experimental intervention among low-income Hispanic women in community health clinics. *Health Education & Behavior, 38*(5), 452-461, doi: 10.1177/1090198110375037

Dent, R., Trudeau, M., Pritchard, K. I., Hanna, W. M., Kahn, H. K., Sawka, C. A., Narod, S. A. (2007). Triple-negative breast cancer: Clinical features and patterns of recurrence. *Clinical*

Cancer Research, 13(15 Pt 1), 4429-4434. doi: 10.1158/1078-0432.CCR-06-3045

Dickson-Swift, V., James, E. L., Kippen, S., & Liamputton, P. (2007). Doing sensitive research: what challenges do qualitative researchers face? *Qualitative Research, 7*; 327. doi: dx.doi.org/10.1177/1468794107078515.

Draper, A. A., & Swift, J. A. (2011). Qualitative research in nutrition and dietetics: data collection issues. Journal Of Human Nutrition & Dietetics, 24(1), 3-12. doi:10.1111/j.1365-277X.2010.01117.x

Feldman, E. J. (1981). *A practical guide to the conduct of field research in the social sciences.* Boulder, CO: Westview Press.

Fishbein, M., & Ajzen, A. (1975). *Belief, attitude, intention, and behavior.* New York, NY: Wiley.

Freeman, H. P. (2003). Commentary on the meaning of race in science and society. *Cancer Epidemiology, Biomarkers and Prevention, 12*, 232s-236s. Retrieved from http://cebp.aacrjournals.org/content/12/3/232s.shorthttp://cebp.aacrjournals.org/content/12/3/232s.shorthttp://cebp.aacrjournals.org/content/12/3/232s.shorthttp://cebp.aacrjournals.org/content/12/3/232s.short

Frisby, C. M. (2012). Messages of hope: Health communication strategies that address barriers preventing Black women from screening for breast cancer. *Cancer, 32*(5), 489–505. doi: 10.1177/0021934702032005 01

Gehlert, S., & Coleman, R. (2010). Using community-based participatory research to ameliorate cancer disparities. *Health & Social Work, 35*(4), 302-309. doi: 10.1093/hsw/35.4.302

Gierisch, M. J., O'Neill, S. C., Rimer, B. K., DeFrank, J. T., Bowling, J. M., & Skinner, S. C. (2009). Factors associated with annual-interval mammography for women in their 40s. *Cancer Epidemiology, 33*, 72–78. doi: 10.1016/j.cdp.2009.03.001

Glesne, C. (2011). Becoming qualitative researchers: An introduction (4th Ed.). Boston: Pearson

Green, L. W., & Kreuter, M. W. (2005). *Health program planning: An educational and ecological approach* (4th ed.). New York, NY: McGraw-Hill.

Greer-Williams, N. J., Enoch, K. S., Booth, B., Starlard-Davenport, A., Sarto, G. E., & Kieber-Emmons, T. (2014). Rural African American women and breast cancer: social determinants of health shape accessibility to conceptualize health in the Arkansas Delta. *Journal Of Rural & Community Development, 9*(2), 51-66.

Gullatte, M. M., Brawley, O., Kinney, A., Powe, B., & Mooney, K. (2010). Religiosity, spirituality, and cancer fatalism beliefs on delay in breast cancer diagnosis in African American women. *Journal of Religion and Health, 49*(1), 62–72. doi: 10.1007/s10943-008-9232-8

Hardin, A. H. (2012). Fear as a barrier in mammography screenings. *Kaleidoscope, 10*, Article 10. Retrieved from

http://uknowledge.uky.edu/cgi/viewcontent.cgi?
article=1057 &context=kaleidoscope

Hatcher-Keller, J., Rayens, M. K., Dignan, M., Schoenberg, N., &
Allison, P. (2014). Beliefs regarding mammography screening
among women visiting the emergency department for nonurgent
care. *Journal of Emergency Nursing, 40*(2), 27-35. doi:
10.1016/j.jen.2013.01.015

Heiney, S. P. (2014). Social disconnection in African American women
with breast cancer. *Oncology Nursing Forum, 41*(1), E28-E34.
doi:10.1188/14.ONF.E28-E34

Heisey, R., Clemons, M., Granek, L., Fergus, K., Hum, S., Lord, B., . .
. Fitzgerald, B. (2011). Health care strategies to promote earlier
presentation of symptomatic breast cancer: perspectives of
women and family physicians. *Current Oncology, 18*(5), e277-
e237. doi: 10.3747/co.v18i5.869

Hochbaum, G. M. (1958). *Public participation in medical screening
programs: A socio-psychological study* (PHS Publication No.
572). Washington, DC: Government Printing Office.

Hoffman, H. J., LaVerda, N. L., Levine, P. H., Young, H. A.,
Alexander, L. M., Patierno, S. R., & the District of Columbia
Citywide Patient Navigator Research Program Research Group.
(2011). Having health insurance does not eliminate
race/ethnicity-associated delays in breast cancer diagnosis in the
District of Columbia. *Cancer, 117*(16), 3824-3832. doi:
10.1002/cncr.25970

House, J. S., Umberson, D., & Landis, K. R. (1998). Structures and processes of social support. *Annual Review of Sociology, 14*, 293-318. doi: 10.1146/annurev.so.14.080188.001453

Howlader, N., Noone, A. M., Krapcho, M., Garshell, J., Neyman, N., Altekruse, S. F., . Cronin, K. A. (Eds.). (2013). *SEER cancer statistics review, 1975-2010*. Bethesda, MD: National Cancer Institute. Retrieved from http://seer.cancer.gov/csr/1975_2011/

Hughes, D. (2013). Majority of women lack accurate knowledge of their own breast cancer risk. *Chemotherapy Advisor.* Retrieved from http://www.chemotherapyadvisor.com/majority-of-women-lack-accurate-knowledge-of-their-own-breast-cancer-risk/article/310898/

Jemal, A., Murray, T., Ward, E., Samuels, A., Tiwari, R. C., Ghafoor, A., . . . Thun, M. J. (2005). Cancer statistics, 2005. *CA: A Cancer Journal for Clinicians, 55*, 10-30. doi: 10.3322/canjclin.55.1.10

Kadivar, H., Goff, B. A., Phillips, W. R., Andrilla, C. H., Berg, A. O., & Baldwin, L. M. (2012). Non-recommended breast and colorectal cancer screening for young women: A vignette-based survey. *American Journal of Preventative Medicine, 43*(3), 231-239. doi: 10.1016/j.amepre.2012.05.022

Katzung B. G., Masters S. B., & Trevor A. J. (2009). *Basic & clinical pharmacology* (11th ed.). New York, NY: McGraw-Hill Medical.

Kaur, P., Nagaraja, G. M., Zheng, H., Gizachew, D., Galukande, M.,

Krishnan, S., & Asea, A. (2012). A mouse model for triple-negative breast cancer tumor-initiating cells (TNBC-TICs) exhibits similar aggressive phenotype to the human disease. *BMC Cancer, 12*, 120. doi: 10.1186/1471-2407-12-120

Khaliq, W., Visvanathan, K., Landis, R., & Wright, S. M. (2013). Breast cancer screening preferences among hospitalized Women. *Journal Of Women's Health 22*(7), 637-642. doi:10.1089/jwh.2012.4083

King, N., & Horrocks, C. (2010). Interviews in Qualitative Research. Thousand Oaks, CA: Sage.

Kingsley, C. (2010, March). Cultural and socioeconomic factors affecting cancer screening, early detection and care in the Latino population. Retrieved from Ethnomed website: http://ethnomed.org/clinical /cancer/cultural-and-socioeconomic-factors-affecting-cancer-screening-early-detection-and-care-in-the-latino-population

Komenaka, I. K., Martinez, M. E., Pennington, R. E., Jr., Hsu, C. H., Clare, S. E., Thompson, P. A., . . . Goulet, R. J., Jr. (2010). Race and ethnicity and breast cancer outcomes in an underinsured population. *Journal of the National Cancer Institute, 102*(15), 1178-1187. doi: 10.1093/jnci/djq215

Lauver, D., Settersen, L., Kane, J. H. & Henrique, J. B. (2003). Tailored messages, external barriers, and women's utilization of professional breast cancer screening overtime. American Cancer Society, 2724-2735.

Lin, R., & Plevritis, S. (2012). Comparing the benefits of screening for
breast cancer and lung cancer using a novel natural history
model. *Cancer Causes & Control, 23*(1), 175-185. doi:
10.1007/s10552-011-9866-9

Lincoln, Y., S, & Guba, E., G. (1985). Naturalistic Inquiry. Newbury
Park, CA: Sage Publications. ISBN: 0803924313

Lukwago, S. N., Kreuter, M. W., Holt, C. L., Steger-May, K.,
Bucholz, D. C. & Skinner, C. S. (2003). Sociocultural correlates
of breast cancer knowledge and screening in urban African
American women. *American Journal of Public Health, 93*(80),
1271-1274.

Lund, M. J., Triver, K. F., Porter, P. L., Coates, R. J., Leyland-Jones,
B., Brawley, O. W., Eley, J. W. (2009). Race and triple negative
threats to breast cancer survival: A population-based study in
Atlanta, GA. *Breast Cancer Research and Treatment, 113,* 357–
370. doi: 10.1007/s10549-008-9926-3

Lynn, B., Yoo, G. J., & Levine, E. G. (2013). Trust in the Lord:
Religious and spiritual practices of African American breast
cancer survivors. *Journal of Religion and Health.* Advance
online publication. doi: 10.1007/s10943-013-9750-x

Manski, R., Moeller, J., Chen, H., Schimmel, J., St. Clair, P., & Pepper,
J. (2013). Patterns of older Americans' health care utilization
over time. *American Journal Of Public Health, 103*(7), 1314-
1324. doi: 10.2105/AJPH.2012.301124

Marchick, J., & Henson, D. E. (2005). Correlations between access to

mammography and breast cancer stage at diagnosis. *Cancer,*
103, 1571–1580. doi: 10.2105/AJPH.2012.301124

Marshall, M. N. (1996). Sampling for qualitative research. *Family*
Practice, 13(6), 522–526. doi:10.1093/fampra/13.6.522

Masi, C. M., & Gehlert, S. (2009). Perception of breast cancer
treatment among African-American women and men:
Implications for interventions. *Journal of General Internal*
Medicine, 24(3), 408-414. doi: 10.1007/s11606-008-0868-6

Mason, M. (2010). Sample Size and Saturation in PhD Studies Using
Qualitative Interviews. *Forum: Qualitative Social Research,*
11(3). Retrieved from http://www.qualitative-
research.net/index.php/fqs/article/view/1428/3027

McQueen, A., Kreuter, M. W., Kalesan, B., & Alcaraz, K. I. (2011).
Understanding narrative effects: The impact of breast cancer
survivor stories on message processing, attitudes and beliefs
among African American women. *Health Psychology, 30*(6),
674-682. doi: 10.1037/a0025395

Menashe, I., Anderson, W. F., Jatoi, I., & Rosenberg, P. S. (2009).
Underlying causes of the Black-European American racial
disparity in breast cancer mortality: A population-based
analysis. *Journal of the National Cancer Institute, 101*(14),
993-1000. doi: 10.1093/jnci/djp176

Mooradian, A. D. (2010. Barriers related to mammography use for
breast cancer screening among minority women. Journal of
National Medical Association, 102(3):206-18.

Mousavi, S. M., Försti, A., Sundquist, K., & Hemminki, K. (2013). Do reproductive factors influence T, N, and M classes of ductal and lobular breast cancers? A nation-wide follow-up study. *Plos ONE, 8*(5), 1-10. doi:10.1371/journal.pone.0058867

National Institutes of Health, National Cancer Institute. (2008). Cancer health disparities. Retrieved from http://www.cancer.gov/cancertopics/factsheet/disparities/cancer-health-disparities.

National Institutes of Health, National Cancer Institute. (2013). Breast cancer. Retrieved from http://www.cancer.gov/cancertopics/types/breast

Nelson, H. D., Tyne, K., Naik, A., Bougatsos, C., Chan, B. K., & Humphrey, L. (2009). Screening for breast cancer: An update for the U.S. Preventive Services Task Force. *Annals of Internal Medicine, 151*(10), 727–737. doi: 10.7326/0003-4819-151-10-200911170-00009

Nofech-Mozes, S., Trudeau, M., Kahn, H. K., Dent, R., Rawlinson, E., Sun, P., . . . Hanna, W. M. (2009). Patterns of recurrence in the basal and non-basal subtypes of triple-negative breast cancers. *Breast Cancer Research and Treatment, 118*(1), 131-137. doi: 10.1007/s10549-008-0295-8

Ogedegbe, G., Cassells, A. N., Robinson, C. M., Duhamel, K., Tobin, J. N., Sox, C. H. & Dietrich, A. J. (2005). Perceptions of barriers and facilitators of cancer early detection among low-income minority women in community health centers. Journal of the National Medical Association, 97(2), 162-170

Onitilo, A. A., Engel, J. M., Greenlee, R. T., & Mukesh, B. N. (2009). Breast cancer subtypes based on ER/PR and Her2 expression: Comparison of clinicopathologic features and survival. *Clinical Medicine Research, 7*(1-2), 4-13. doi: 10.3121/cmr.2008.825

Pasick, R. J., & Burke, N. J. (2008). A critical review of theory in breast cancer screening promotion across cultures. *Annual Review of Public Health, 29*, 351-368. doi: 10.1146/annurev.publhealth.29.020907.143420

Patton, M. Q. (2002). *Qualitative research & evaluation methods* (3rd ed.). Thousand Oaks, CA: Sage. Isbn: 9780761919711 Pearson.

Peek, M. E., Sayad, J. V., & Markwardt, R. (2008). Fear, fatalism and breast cancer screening in low-income African-American women: The role of clinicians and the health care system. *Journal of General Internal Medicine, 23*(11), 1847–1853. doi: 10.1007/s11606-008-0756-0

Phillips, J. M., Cohen, M. Z. & Tarzian, A. J. (2001). African American women's experiences with breast cancer screening. Journal of Nursing Scholarship, 33(2), 135-140.

Polite, B. N., & Olopade, O. I. (2005). Breast cancer and race: A rising tide does not lift all boats equally. *Perspectives in Biological Medicine, 48*(1 Suppl), S166–S175. doi: 10.1353/pbm.2005.0041

Prochaska, J. O. (1991). Assessing how people change. Cancer, 67, 805-807. doi: 10.1002/1097-0142(19910201)67:3+<805::AID-CNCR2820671409>3.0.CO;2-4

Prochaska, J. O., Redding, C. A., Harlow, L. L., Rossi, J. S., & Velcier, W. F. (1994). The transtheoretical model of change and HIV prevention: A review. Health Education, 21, 471-486. doi: 10.1177/109019819402100410

Rahman, S., Price, J. H., Dignan, M., Rahman, S., Lindquist, P. S., & Jordan, T. R. (2009). Access to mammography facilities and detection of breast cancer by screening mammography: A GIS approach. *International Journal of Cancer Prevention*, *2*(6), 403-413. Pmid: 20628557

Rakowski, W., Wyn, R., Breen, N., Meissner, H., & Clark, M. A. (2010). Prevalence and correlates of recent and repeat mammography among California women ages 55–79. *Cancer Epidemiology, 34*(2), 168 –177. doi: 10.1016/j.canep.2010.02.005

Research in Psychology, 1, 39-54. doi: 10.1191/1478088704qp004oa

Rice, V. H. (2000). Handbook of Stress, coping, and health: Implications for nursing research and practice. (pp.337-339). London: Sage Publications, Inc. International Educational and Professional Publisher.

Rosenstock, I. M. (1960). What research in motivation suggests for public health. *American Journal of Public Health*, *50*, 295-301. doi: 10.2105/AJPH.50.3_Pt_1.295

RTIPS (2015). Breast Cancer Screening Intervention Programs http://rtips.cancer.gov/rtips/topicPrograms.do?topicId=102263 &choice=default

Russell, K. M., Monahan, P., Wagle, A., & Champion, V. (2006).
Differences in health and cultural beliefs by stage of
mammography screening adoption in African American
Women. *American Cancer Society, 109*(2 Suppl), 386-395.
pmid: 17133417

Sabatino, S. A., Lawrence, B., Elder, R., Mercer, S. L., Wilson, K. M.,
deVinney, B., . . . Community Preventative Services Task
Force. (2012). Effectiveness of interventions to increase
screening for breast, cervical and colorectal cancers. Nine
updated systematic reviews for the guide to community
preventive services. *American Journal of Preventative
Medicine, 43*(1), 97-118. doi: 10.1016/j.amepre.2012.04.009

Sadala, M., Bruzos, G., Pereira, E., & Bucuvic, E. (2012). Patients'
experiences of peritoneal dialysis at home: a phenomenological
approach. Revista Latino-Americana De Enfermagem (RLAE),
20(1), 68-75. doi: 10.1590/S0104-11692012000100010

Sail, K., Franzini, L., Lairson, D., & Du, X. (2012). Differences in
treatment and survival among African-American and Caucasian
women with early stage operable breast cancer. Ethnicity &
Health, 17(3), 309-323. doi:10.1080/13557858.2011.628011

Sante et Services socieaux Quebec. (n.d.) Advantages, limitations or
drawbacks to screening mammograms. Retrieved from
http://www.msss.gouv.qc.ca/sujets
/santepub/pqdcs/index.php?avantages-limites-inconvenients-
mammographie-en.

Sarkissyan, M., Wu, Y., & Vadgama, J. V. (2011). Obesity is
associated with breast cancer in African American women but
not Hispanic women in south Los Angeles. *Cancer, 117*(16),
3814-3823. doi: 10.1002/cncr.25956

Seidman, I. (2006). *Interviewing as qualitative research: A guide for
researchers in education and the social sciences* (3rd ed.). New
York, NY: Teachers College Press. Isbn: 978-0807746660

Shank, G. D. (2006). Qualitative research: A personal skills approach
(2nd ed.). Columbus, OH: Pearson Publishing. Isbn: 978-
0131719491

Sheppard, V. B., Graves, K. D., Christopher, J., Hurtado-de-Mendoza,
A., Talley, C., & Williams, K. P. (2013). African American
women's limited knowledge and experiences with genetic
counseling for hereditary breast cancer. *Journal of Genetic
Counselling. 23*(3), 311-322. doi: 10.1007/s10897-013-9663-6

Shigematsu, H., Nakamura, Y., Tanaka, K., Shiotani, S., Koga, C.,
Kawaguchi, H. . . . Ohno, S. (2010). A case of HER-2-positive
advanced inflammatory breast cancer with invasive
micropapillary component showing a clinically complete
response to concurrent trastuzumab and paclitaxel treatment.
International Journal Of Clinical Oncology, 15(6), 615-620.
doi: 10.1007/s10147-010-0093-2

Simonds, V. W., Colditz, G. A., Rudd, R. E., & Sequest, T. D. (2011).
Cancer screening among Native Americans in California.
Ethnicity & Disease, 21, 202-209. pmid: 21749025

Smith, J.A., & Osborn, M. (2003). Interpretative phenomenological analysis. In J. A. Smith (Ed.), Qualitative psychology: A practical guide to research methods (pp. 51-80). Thousand Oaks, CA: Sage. Isbn: 9780761972310

Smith, G. L., Shih, Y. C., Xu, Y., Giordano, S. H., Smith, B. D., Perkins, G. H., . . . Buchholz, T. A. (2010). Racial disparities in the use of radio-therapy after breast-conserving surgery: A national Medicare study. *Cancer, 116*(3), 734-741. doi: 10.1002/cncr.24741

Smith, J. A., Jarman, M., & Osborn, M. (1999). Doing interpretative phenomenological analysis. In M. Murray & K. Chamberlain (Eds.), Qualitative health psychology: Theories and methods (pp. 218-240). Thousand Oaks, CA: Sage. ISBN: 9780857022028

Smith, J.A. (2004). Reflecting on the development of interpretative phenomenological and its contribution to qualitative research in psychology. Qualitative Research in Psychology, 1(1), 39–54.

Smith, J.A., & Osborn, M. (2003). Interpretative phenomenological analysis. In J. A. Smith (Ed.), Qualitative Psychology: A Practical Guide to Methods (pp. 53-80). London: Sage.

Sotiriou, C., & Pusztai, L. (2009). Gene-expression signatures in breast cancer. *New England Journal of Medicine, 360,* 790–800. doi: 10.1056/NEJMra0801289

Spiegelberg H., (1995). Doing phenomenology: Essays on and in phenomenology. The hague: Martinus Nijhoff.

Subramanian, P., Burhan, A., Pallaveshi, L., & Rudnick, A. (2013).
The experience of patients with schizophrenia treated with
repetitive transcranial magnetic stimulation for auditory
hallucinations. *Case Reports In Psychiatry*, 1-5.
doi:10.1155/2013/183582

Summers, C., Saltzstein, S. L., Blair, S. L., Tsukamoto, T. T., & Sadler,
G. R. (2010). Racial/Ethnic differences in early detection of
breast cancer: A Study of 250,985 cases from the California
Cancer Registry. *Journal Of Women's Health 19*(2), 203-207.
doi:10.1089/jwh.2008.1314

Swan, J., Breen, N., Graubard, B. I., McNeel, T. S., Blackman, D.,
Tangka, F. K., & Ballard-Barbash, R. (2010). Data and trends in
cancer screening in the United States: Results from the 2005
National Health Interview Survey. *Cancer, 116*(20), 4872-4881.
doi: 10.1002/cncr.25215

Swinney, J. E., & Dobal, M. T. (2011). Older African American
women's beliefs, attitudes and behaviors about breast cancer.
Research in Gerontological Nursing, 4(1), 9-18. doi:
10.3928/19404921-20101207-01

Taylor, T. R., Huntley, E. D., Sween, J., Makambi, K., Mellman, T. A,
Williams, C. D., . . . Frederick, W. (2012). An exploratory
analysis of fear of recurrence among African American breast
cancer survivors. *International Journal of Behavioral Medicine,
19*(3), 280-287. doi: 10.1007/s12529-011-9183-4

Tejeda, S., Darnell, J. S., Cho,Y. I., Stolley, M. R., Markossian, T. W.,

& Calhoun, E. A. (2013). Patient barriers to follow-up care for breast and cervical cancer abnormalities. *Journal of Womens Health (Larchmont), 22*(6), 507-517. doi: 10.1089/jwh.2012.3590

Thompson, H. S., Edwards, T., Erwin, D. O., Lee, S. H., Bovbjerg, B., Janforf, L., . . . Romero, J. (2009). Training lay health workers to promote post-treatment breast cancer surveillance in African American breast cancer survivors: Development and implementation of a curriculum. *Journal of Cancer Education, 24*(4), 267-274. doi: 10.1080/08858190902973085

Todd, A., & Stuifbergen, A. (2012). Barriers and facilitators to breast cancer screening: A qualitative study of women with multiple sclerosis. *International Journal of MS Care, 13*(2), 49-56. doi: 10.7224/1537-2073-13.2.49

U.S. Department of Education, Institute of Education Sciences, National Center for Education Statistics. (2008). *Digest of education statistics 2008* (NCES Publication No. 2009-020). Retrieved from http://nces.ed.gov/pubs2009/2009020.pdf

U.S. Department of Health and Human Services, Centers for Disease Control and Prevention. (2012, January 27). Cancer screening – United States, 2010. *Morbidity and Mortality Weekly Report, 61*(3), 41-45.

U.S. Department of Health and Human Services, Centers for Disease Control and Prevention. (2013). Breast cancer. Retrieved from http://www.cdc.gov/cancer/breast/

U.S. Department of Health and Human Services, Centers for Disease Control and Prevention, National Center for Health Statistics. (2010). *Health, United States, 2009 with special feature on medical technology* (DHHS Publication No. 2010-1232). Retrieved from www.cdc.gov/nchs/data/hus/hus09.pdf

U.S. Preventive Services Task Force. (2009). Screening for breast cancer. Retrieved from www.uspreventiveservicestaskforce.org/uspstf/uspsbrca.htm

Umezawa, Y., Lu, Q., You, J., Kagawa-Singer, M., Leake, B., & Maly, R. C. (2012). Belief in divine control, coping and race/ethnicity among older women with breast cancer. *Annals of Behavioral Medicine, 44*(1), 21-32. doi: 10.1007/s12160-012-9358-5

van den Biggelaar, F. J., Kessels, A. G., van Engelshoven, J. M., & Flobbe, K. (2009). Costs and effects of using specialized breast technologists in prereading mammograms in a clinical patient population. *International Journal of Technology Assessment in Health Care, 25*(4), 505-513. doi: 10.1017/S0266462309990377

van Ravesteyn, N. T., Schechter, C. B., Near, A. M., Heijnsdijk, E. A., Stoto, M. A., Draisma, G., . . . Mandelblatt, J. S. (2011). Race-specific impact of natural history, mammography screening, and adjuvant treatment on breast cancer mortality rates in the United States. *Cancer Epidemiol Biomarkers Prev, 20*(1), 112-122. doi: 10.1158/1055-9965.EPI-10-0944

Viswanathan, M., Kraschnewski, J., Nishikawa, B., Morgan, L. C.,

Thieda, P., Honeycutt, A., . . . Jonas, D. (2009). *Outcomes of community health workers interventions* (AHRQ Publication No. 09-E014). Rockville, MD: Agency for Healthcare Research and Quality. Retrieved from http://www.ahrq.gov/research/findings/evidence-based-reports/comhwork-evidence-report.pdf

Vona-Davis, L., Rose, D. P., Hazard, H., Howard-McNatt, M., Adkins, F., Partin, J., & Hobbs, G. (2008). Triple-negative breast cancer and obesity in a rural Appalachian population. *Cancer Epidemiology, Biomarkers & Prevention,17*, 3319–3324. doi: 10.1158/1055-9965.EPI-08-0544

Walker, J. L., (2012).The use of saturation in qualitative research. Canadian Journal of Cardiovascular Nursing Spring; 22(2):37-46. Retrieved from http://connection.ebscohost.com/c/articles/74981872/research-column-use-saturation-qualitative-research

European American , D., Oelke, N. D., & Friesen, S. (2012). Management of a Large Qualitative Data Set: Establishing Trustworthiness of the Data. International Journal Of Qualitative Methods, 11(3), 244-258. Retrieved from http://ejournals.library.ualberta.ca/index.php/IJQM/article/view/9883

Yoo, J. H., Kreuter, M. W., Lai, C., & Fu, Q. (2013). Understanding narrative effects: The role of discrete negative emotions on message processing and attitudes among low-income African

American women. *Health Communication, 29*(5), 494-504. doi: 10.1080/10410236.2013.776001

Young, R. F., Schwartz, K., & Booza, J. (2011). Medical barriers to mammography screening of African American women in a high cancer mortality area: Implications for cancer educators and health providers. *Journal of Cancer Education, 26*(2), 262-269. doi: 10.1007/s13187-010-0184-9

Zhang, L. R., Chiarelli, A. M., Glendon, G., Mirea, L., Knigh, J A., Andrulis, I. L., & Ritvo, P. (2012). Worry is good for breast cancer screening: A study of female relatives from Ontario site of the Breast Cancer Family Registry. *Journal of Cancer Epidemiology, 2012*, Article ID 545062. doi:10.1155/2012/545062

Zollinger, T. W., Champion, V. L., Monahan, P. O., Steele-Moses, S. K., Ziner, K. W., Zhao, Q., . . . Russell, K. M. (2010). Effects of personal characteristics on African American women's beliefs about breast cancer. *American Journal of Health Promotion, 24*(6), 371-377. doi: 10.4278/ajhp.07031727

Appendix A:
Informed Consent

Barriers to Breast Cancer Prevention and Screening among African American Women

You are invited to participate in a research study of barriers to breast cancer prevention and screening among African American Women. You are invited as a possible participant. The inclusion criteria are (a) African American females 40 years of age or older (b) ability to communicate in English language effectively (c) no previous or resent diagnosis of breast cancer within your community (d) participants will be African American women who are willing to share their professed personal barriers, stereotype, socio-economic status, culture, attitudes, beliefs, and how these factors may influence breast cancer screening. Please read this form and ask any questions you may have before acting on this invitation to be in the study. The purpose of this study is to better understand the perceptions of African American women and how these factors may influence breast cancer screening. If you agree to participate in this study, you will be asked to participate in an interview approximately 60 minute in length. The interview location will be in a private room where confidentiality and identity will be kept private at the church or mutually agreed upon location. The interview will be recorded and each interview will be transcribed in coded format to protect the identity of each participate. For example, names will not be used, but coded as Participant1 [P1], Participant2 [P2], etc.; thus, transcript will protect the individual's identity. Each participant will have an opportunity to review the transcript related to their and verify accuracy of her comments. This Member Check Step will validate the credibility of the participant's interview content. Your participation in this study is strictly voluntary. Your decision whether or not to participate will not affect your current or future relations with Worthington Seventh-Day Adventist Church. There are minimal risks associated with participating in this study. The potential benefits of participating in this study may help in understanding the perceived barriers for breast cancer screening among African American Women, how awareness of breast cancer screening and prevention can be promoted among African American women and how stereotype and culture influence African American women's beliefs and behavior in regard to breast cancer screening and prevention. In the event you experience stress or anxiety during your participation in the study you may terminate your participation at any time. You may refuse to answer any questions you consider invasive or stressful. There is no form of compensation for participation. The records of this study will be kept private. Research records will be kept in a locked cabinet; only the researcher will have access to the records. Interviews will be audio recorded for purposes of providing accurate description of your experience. In the event that any report of this study might be published, the researcher will not include any information that will disclose your identity. This study is being conducted by doctoral student at Walden university under the leadership of Dr. Diane Cortner If you have any questions feel free to ask now or contact me at (614) 306-6447, abosede.obikunle@waldenu.edu. The Research Participant Advocate at Walden University is Leilani Endicot; you may contact her at 612-312-1210 or email her at IRB@waldenu.edu if you have questions about your participation in this study. You will receive a copy of this form from the researcher. Walden University's approval number for this study is 05-12-15-0231648 and it expires May 11, 2016.

Statement of Consent: I have read the above information. I have asked questions and received answers. I consent to participate in the study.

Printed Name of Participant

____

Signature Date ____

Signature of
Investigator____

Date ____

Appendix B:
Interview Protocol

Interview Protocol

Date: _______________________________

Interview location: _____________________________

Name of Interviewer____

Name of Interviewee

____

1. How would you describe your family of origin?

2. What do you understand by breast cancer prevention and screening?

3. What concerns do you have about locating and participating in breast cancer screening?

4. How does your awareness level about breast cancer screening influence your utilization of the available screening resources?

5. What are your personal barriers that have influenced your breast cancer screening behavior?

6. Do you see culture and stereotype as barriers to breast cancer screening? (If so, in what ways)

7. What is your attitude and beliefs towards breast cancer screening?

8. How knowledgeable are you about breast cancer screening recommendations? Please explain

9. What are the resources available in your community for breast cancer screening?

10. Do you know how to get available breast cancer screenings? Please describe the process.

11. Have you ever had breast cancer screening? Please explain what type of screening you had and your experience.

12. What was the most challenging aspect of breast cancer screening?

13. What factors in your opinion would better enhance your experience and/or utilization of breast cancer screening?

14. Are you employed and how would you describe your socio-economic status?

15. Does your socio-economic status influence your breast cancer screening habits?

16. Do you have health insurance? If no why and if yes, what does your insurance cover?

17. What type of health insurance do you have if applicable?

18. How affordable is your health insurance, and what factor or factors determined your choice of insurance?

19. How adequate do you think your health insurance is when compared to your health needs

20. What is your advice for African American women about breast cancer screening?

21. What advice do you have for healthcare providers to improve breast cancer screening services for African American women?

Appendix C:
Recruitment Flyer

VOLUNTEERS:

African American females 40 years of age or older

Voluntary Participation in a Doctoral Research Study on Your

Perception of Barriers to Breast Cancer Prevention and Screening

among African American Women

Location: At Your Church

Participation requires an interview for approximately 60 minutes in

length

I appreciate your potential interest in helping with this Study!

Please email abosede.obikunle@waldenu.edu or call (614) 306-6447.

THANKS!

Appendix D:

Observation Guide

Participant #_________________

Based on observations: the following was noted

	Present/Relaxed/ Friendly/Engaged/Interested	Absent/Uncomfortable/ Unfriendly/Abrupt/Uninterested	Comment
Eye Contact			
Body Language			
Tone of Voice			
Answers to Questions			
Attitude			

Table 9. Observation Table

Appendix E:
Interview Time span data

Interview Time span data

Participant 1

Time span	Content Question	Answer
1	2:40.8 - 2:57.4	How would you describe your family of origin?	Born and raised in Africa having lived in USA for many years she lumped into the group of African Americans
2	2:57.4 - 4:17.0	What do you understand by breast cancer prevention and screening?	Personal understanding: prevention comes from awareness, might be genetic but lifestyle pulls the gun, comes from education
3	4:17.0 - 4:48.8		empowering of women
4	4:48.8 - 7:16.7	What concerns do you have about locating and participating in	Concern: I would love to participate but I love education women, the most concern is on

		breast cancer screening?	education
5	7:16.7 - 9:32.4	How does your awareness level about breast cancer screening influence your utilization of the available screening resources?	believe that the screenings not very healthy, screening is painful
6	10:13.2 - 11:37.4		seem to me that the exposition in screening may cause cancer
7	11:37.4 - 13:17.3	What are your personal barriers that have influenced your breast cancer screening behavior?	My knowledge in natural health care makes me have my preferences when it comes to breast cancer screening
8	13:17.3 - 16:13.2	Do you see culture and stereotype as barriers to breast cancer screening? (If so, in what ways)	Culture may influence screening be in terms of poverty and lack of education. Exposure to rights and privileges women don't feel like going to hospital because they feel it's not necessary unless they become very ill. preventive measures are

			not part of the culture
9	16:13.2 - 18:17.2		stereotype plays a role because some think it is genetic and think they can do nothing about it
10	18:17.2 - 24:10.0	What is your attitude and beliefs towards breast cancer screening?	Breast cancer screening is an effort towards the right direction, but more education and preventive measures should be given is not taken seriously because it doesn't really make a lot of money
11	24:10.0 - 25:46.7	How knowledgeable are you about breast cancer screening recommendations? Please explain	Very knowledgeable. Government expects yearly mammogram, take exams as regularly as possible
12	25:46.7 - 26:59.3	What are the resources available in your community for breast cancer screening?	There are free mammograms in some clinics for people. it is displayed that hospitals have free mammograms
13	26:59.3 - 29:04.0	Do you how to get available breast cancer	I don't think I might be correct in the procedure

		screenings? Please describe the process.	because I have not taken one in a long time
14	29:04.0 - 29:30.5	Have you ever had breast cancer screening? Please explain what type of screening you had and your experience.	I have participated
15	29:30.5 - 30:17.0	What was the most challenging aspect of breast cancer screening?	most challenging aspect was very painful because of the pressing
16	30:17.0 - 31:22.9	What factors in your opinion would better enhance your experience and/or utilization of breast cancer screening?	more education as to the effects of breast cancer on a Woman's life would enhance the utilization of screening
17	31:22.9 - 32:58.5	Are you employed and how would you describe your socio-economic status?	Not employed, work for myself. socio-economic status not very great
18	32:58.5 - 33:47.6	Does your socio-economic status	socio-economic status does affect screening

		influence your breast cancer screening habits?	habits
19	33:47.6 - 34:36.4	Do you have health insurance? If no why and if yes, what does your insurance cover?	Obama health care insurance, don't know what it covers
20	33:53.3 - 35:39.9	How affordable is your health insurance, and what factor or factors determined your choice of insurance?	choice of insurance determined by being compulsory at the state of California to avoid penalty
21	35:39.9 - 36:21.0	How adequate do you think your health insurance is when compared to your health needs	don't have any particular health need
22	36:21.0 - 37:50.5	What is your advice for African American women about breast cancer screening?	advice would be for African American women to be more pro active and take up the available resources to them
23	37:50.5 - 41:58.0	What advice do you have for healthcare	advice for health care providers to start

			looking at the causes rather than healing and help people know what is available to them
24	41:58.0 - 44:05.5	Other Comments	finance issue should play a role, family support

Participant 2

	Time span	**Content Question**	**Answer**
25	45:09.0 - 46:23.0	How would you describe your family of origin?	From Africa
26	46:23.0 - 47:36.6	What do you understand by breast cancer prevention and screening?	Breast cancer prevention and screening. Education and awareness is the most important thing, self-breast examination, monthly routine self-breast examination. Going to the doctor and radiology regularly. everybody can be involved no matter the genetics

27	48:18.1 - 50:01.6		It is important that everybody has health care insurance. has insurance, sees the doctor twice a year, people without insurance have health challenges
28	50:01.6 - 50:42.8	What concerns do you have about locating and participating in breast cancer screening?	no problem with finding and participating screening because it has become a routine since the last two years
29	56:45.4 - 56:47.1	How does your awareness level about breast cancer screening influence your utilization of the available screening resources?	knowledge that she should do it twice every year she calls the doctor
30	56:45.4 - 56:47.7	What are your personal barriers that have influenced your breast cancer screening behavior?	Initially to be fiddling with herself and massaging her breasts didn't really make sense to her. As years passed she learnt that it was a wise thing to do

31	57:51.4 - 59:52.5	Do you see culture and stereotype as barriers to breast cancer screening? (If so, in what ways)	Culture and stereotype: yes, fiddling with self. Culture does not allow a woman to be playing with herself like that, Understand to change are there and they don't want to change. they feel that it is not necessary but with education it can improve
32	59:52.5 - 1:01:02.7	What is your attitude and beliefs towards breast cancer screening?	Breast cancer screening has helped identify breast cancer at an early age. screening should be encouraged and awareness introduced through education continued
33	1:01:02.7 - 1:02:30.7	How knowledgeable are you about breast cancer screening recommendations? Please explain	She knows check themselves out, see doctors, schedule yearly mammogram after certain age, and follow up. She thinks it is good enough. Some people have to chuck a few dollars. The amount you put there can't be compared with benefits

34	1:02:30.7 - 1:04:41.8	What are the resources available in your community for breast cancer screening?	Free breast cancer screening. Even people who don't have insurance can get screening. Insurances are there to cover. A lot of community effort to ensure women has screening.
35	1:04:41.8 - 1:06:08.9	Do you how to get available breast cancer screenings? Please describe the process.	She knows how to get screening. Some organizations have free screening. Some people tell you to find a doctor if they don't have their own doctors with the reports. Unless one is not interested. those who are interested ask questions
36	1:06:08.9 - 1:08:16.5	Have you ever had breast cancer screening? Please explain what type of screening you had and your experience.	She has had screening. She does self-examination, she goes to the doctor. she has had mammogram, which she paid for initially but insurance

37	1:08:16.5 - 1:09:35.5	What was the most challenging aspect of breast cancer screening?	When she did not have an appointment in time. It took 3 months to see a doctor, but that was not a problem. the screening makes her feel that she is okay and makes her relaxed and can move forward
38	1:09:35.5 - 1:11:18.8	What factors in your opinion would better enhance your experience and/or utilization of breast cancer screening?	she is okay
39	1:11:18.8 - 1:12:12.1	Are you employed and how would you describe your socio-economic status?	Employed, work full time waiting for retirement in a couple of years, she has children some in college but do not have a problem really
40	1:12:12.1 - 1:12:54.0	Does your socio-economic status influence your breast cancer screening habits?	She has education and awareness and teaches it. no challenge

41	1:12:54.0 - 1:13:59.8	Do you have health insurance? If no why and if yes, what does your insurance cover?	She has insurance cover. Breast health examination screening. Dental covered. Regular insurance. Obama care
42	1:13:59.8- 1:15:22.8	How affordable is your health insurance, and what factor or factors determined your choice of insurance?	Insurance is as per income and they have to adjust and make it work. It's working. only concern is if it will cover breast health eyes, dental, I don't have a lot of health challenges
43	1:15:22.8 - 1:15:47.7	How adequate do you think your health insurance is when compared to your health needs	I make use of the health insurance. She doesn't have health challenges. health insurance is adequate
44	1:15:47.7 - 1:16:20.4	What is your advice for African American women about breast cancer screening?	Advise them to breast screening. Self-examination is most important. Water therapy. Use of water washing up. Watching up with doctors. It's not that you must place yourself as a sick

			person to get attention. It is important to ensure you have adequate health. Utilize what you have in the community what you can do naturally for yourself. Food wise, physically, hydro therapy to help you keep in shape. Do screening and check yourself up as needed. It doesn't hurt. some of them are less
45	1:16:20.4 - 1:16:45.2	What advice do you have for healthcare providers to improve breast cancer screening services for African American women?	Education. Most times problems came up because they don't know. Education, information, creating awareness. Tell them when they are healthy.
46	1:16:45.2 - 1:17:22.3	Other Comments	Health is wealth and it is a privilege which they can create and help put into place. They have a duty to humanity to live their part. My family had breast cancer, m----had breast cancer. I can change my DNA by doing what

they did not do right.
orientation, education,
creating awareness

Participant 3

	Time span	Content Question	Answer
1	0:00.0 - 1:30.6	How would you describe your family of origin?	From Africa, Nigeria. citizens of USA
2	1:30.6 - 2:40.9	What do you understand by breast cancer prevention and screening?	Mammogram screening is very common in women when you notice a lump in the breast you go to the doctor quickly and the doctor will send you to mammogram and if it is positive you go to surgery. examine the breast every day and if you feel that there is something wrong with it you go find a doctor
3	2:40.9 - 5:02.3	What concerns do you have about locating and participating in breast cancer screening?	There are places where screening is done. Look online, ask a doctor or go hospitals, sometimes on TV they try to educate, no issues about locating. No problems in participating. If there is any weird it is good to participate it

			is better for one to go in time to know whether you have it or not. it is good to be knowledgeable about the breast cancer and the body to do the test, no concerns
4	5:02.3 - 6:10.1	How does your awareness level about breast cancer screening influence your utilization of the available screening resources?	Any time she goes to the doctor's visit she is given some pamphlets, in TV, and radio. Sure she does the screening. high level
5	6:10.1 - 7:58.9	What are your personal barriers that have influenced your breast cancer screening behavior?	No barrier. as soon as it is time to go to screening she does it, nothing stops her
6	7:58.9 - 9:33.2	Do you see culture and stereotype as barriers to breast cancer screening? (If so, in what ways)	Before the advent of civilization. touching your breast is not a good thing
7	9:33.2 - 10:37.8	What is your attitude and beliefs towards	Positive attitude to anything that makes her live longer, no opposition to screening. she

		breast cancer screening?	beliefs it should be done
8	10:37.8 - 11:34.2	How knowledgeable are you about breast cancer screening recommendations? Please explain	very knowledgeable
9	11:34.2 - 12:09.4	What are the resources available in your community for breast cancer screening?	most important thing in the community they put posters trying to tell where you can go for screening, pass information, tell them notices about where to go and what to do
10	12:09.4 - 13:09.7	Do you how to get available breast cancer screenings? Please describe the process.	when she goes to the center where she does the screening, she is explained to what she is going to do and given material to wear and she is directed to the mammogram machine
11	13:09.7 - 15:03.4	Have you ever had breast cancer screening? Please explain what type of screening you had and your experience.	She has done mammogram before. About 20 times, good experience. The machine presses the breasts and she can see her breasts on the screen although she does not know how to interpret. no discomfort

12	15:03.4 - 15:50.5	What was the most challenging aspect of breast cancer screening?	. afraid of what could happen
13	15:50.5 - 17:06.1	What factors in your opinion would better enhance your experience and/or utilization of breast cancer screening?	sophisticated equipment nowadays makes her happy that there is opportunity to screen,
14	17:06.1 - 18:18.7	Are you employed and how would you describe your socio-economic status?	Not employed but retired. she is good
15	18:18.7 - 19:15.9	Does your socio-economic status influence your breast cancer screening habits?	social economic status does not affect screening
16	19:15.9 - 19:38.7	Do you have health insurance? If no why and if yes, what does your insurance cover?	Health insurance. full insurance Medicare and medicate, Molina is health provider, Covers all her health needs

17	19:38.7 - 20:35.3	How affordable is your health insurance, and what factor or factors determined your choice of insurance?	low income earner the state takes responsibility of the insurance
18	20:35.3 - 21:37.6	How adequate do you think your health insurance is when compared to your health needs	
19	21:37.6 - 22:39.2	What is your advice for African American women about breast cancer screening?	Advice on African American: going for screening is okay. should try to do self examination to check for any pain or any lump
20	22:39.2 - 23:47.9	What advice do you have for healthcare providers to improve breast cancer screening services for African American women?	Make it twice a year.
21	23:47.9	Other Comments	have group discussions too for

| | | more learning about breast cancer screening |

Participant 4

	Time span	**Content Question**	**Answer**
	- 26:26.0		more learning about breast cancer screening
1	0:00.0 - 2:12.3	How would you describe your family of origin?	Originate in America. born in the south Mississippi
2	2:12.3 - 3:07.5	What do you understand by breast cancer prevention and screening?	Self examination and breast screening to detect early breast cancer. Screening is fearful. once you have detected breast cancer is fearful
3	3:07.5 - 6:10.4	What concerns do you have about locating and participating in breast cancer screening?	I don't like screening because it is painful, fearful of breast cancer detection. Doesn't do regular because of the fear. 62 years old and has only done it twice. Went to doctor's office for screening. Equipment and screening was very painful. Put on the machine and squeeze. She does self examination.
4	6:10.4 - 8:26.1	How does your awareness level	Instead of mammogram does self examination. Wouldn't go

		about breast cancer screening influence your utilization of the available screening resources?	for mammogram. She wouldn't go for mammogram for fear of positive result. its better she does not know
5	8:26.1 - 11:02.2	What are your personal barriers that have influenced your breast cancer screening behavior?	Family members have had breast cancer and it was detected early and the process she went through she does not want to go through that. Losing hair is most challenging and she loves people. find it extremely painful and breasts easily bruise and very ticklish she wouldn't want to be touched by anyone else
6	11:02.2 - 19:40.5	Do you see culture and stereotype as barriers to breast cancer screening? (If so, in what ways)	Doesn't think culture contributes to any behavior. She wouldn't take the treatment because she thinks she has lived her life and would live it for someone else. Causes of breast cancer may have come from nourishing babies for European American people. Most African American women do not do self examination or go to screening. African American uses their hands more than the European American women do.

7	19:40.5 - 21:21.6	What is your attitude and beliefs towards breast cancer screening?	There must be a different better way for breast screening other than mammogram. the screening process is most challenging, the way the breasts are handled
8	21:21.6 - 22:56.2	How knowledgeable are you about breast cancer screening recommendations? Please explain	Knowledge is good; she has been in the medical field for a long time. however, following them is the issue
9	22:56.2 - 23:55.8	What are the resources available in your community for breast cancer screening?	Free breast screening at different places. There is no time you can't go for breast screening. there has never a reason for having breast screening if you want it
10	23:55.8 - 25:07.2	Do you how to get available breast cancer screenings? Please describe the process.	In the health clinic there are flyers and you can ask the doctor even if you had gone there for anything else.
11	25:07.2 - 26:27.7	Have you ever had breast cancer screening? Please explain what type	Have had a mammogram. She felt that she was being handled too much; there was pain, sores, and bruises. she did not like it

		of screening you had and your experience.	
12	26:27.7 - 27:24.9	What was the most challenging aspect of breast cancer screening?	Being there, never wanted to know, never wanted to know the outcome. To go again never. she had the last screening ten years when she was in her fifties the first one when she was in her forties
13	27:24.9 - 31:33.4	What factors in your opinion would better enhance your experience and/or utilization of breast cancer screening?	Elimination of some of the presses, the toleration the touch. The equipment should be improved. The procedures of pressing and touching, the way the machine compresses. instruct the woman where to place where to touch, how to handle the machine
14	31:33.4 - 33:26.7	Are you employed and how would you describe your socio-economic status?	Employed. Not a rich but makes a decent living. She manages; she can help her children and grand children and can retire if she wants. she can take care of her needs
15	33:26.7 - 34:20.3	Does your socio-economic status influence your	It does not. she can get what she needs

		breast cancer screening habits?	
16	34:20.3 - 35:02.6	Do you have health insurance? If no why and if yes, what does your insurance cover?	Yes. Covers all her medical expenses at the point that it is at minimal.
17	35:02.6 - 35:27.8		Med life insurance. Does not have older health insurance.
18	35:27.8 - 36:08.9	How affordable is your health insurance, and what factor or factors determined your choice of insurance?	med life is for the company that she works for and it is affordable, comfortable with it
19	36:08.9 - 36:43.7	How adequate do you think your health insurance is when compared to your health needs	Adequacy is good. She doesn't take medication for anything she does not go to the doctor regularly. covers her health needs
20	36:43.7 - 37:37.5	What is your advice for African American women	Encourage them to have screening. by all means have mammogram and do self examination

	Time span	Question	Answer
		about breast cancer screening?	
21	37:37.5 - 38:27.4	What advice do you have for healthcare providers to improve breast cancer screening services for African American women?	Please eliminate some of the equipment. Don't handle so much of the breasts. Make the woman anticipate more on the touching and pressing. eliminate pain
22	38:27.4 - 40:09.7	Other Comments	the cost of screening, the process of having cancer is the greatest fear

Participant 5

	Time span	Content Question	Answer
1	0:00.0 - 3:21.3	How would you describe your family of origin?	Father African America, mother Indian America. grew up in North Carolina
2	3:21.3 - 6:33.5	What do you understand by breast cancer prevention and screening?	Very important to be screened for all health issues and especially for breast cancer screening. She does yearly mammogram at the

			mammogram center. Husband does her examination per month and he knows what he is doing. he thinks it is fun
3	6:33.5 - 7:25.4	What concerns do you have about locating and participating in breast cancer screening?	I have been able to have screening within my own community
4	7:25.4 - 8:52.2	How does your awareness level about breast cancer screening influence your utilization of the available screening resources?	Its more comfortable knowing that the resources are there, there are even mobile units for those who cannot go to the center
5	8:52.2 - 10:39.2	What are your personal barriers that have influenced your breast cancer screening behavior?	Doing well in that regard
6	10:39.2 - 11:20.6	Do you see culture and stereotype as barriers to breast	Some African America women feel they don't feel that they need to have to see

7	11:20.6 - 12:09.5	What is your attitude and beliefs towards breast cancer screening?	It's much needed. although that she is very spiritual they need to know they are in 21st century and take up available resources
8	12:09.5 - 13:41.5	How knowledgeable are you about breast cancer screening recommendations? Please explain	She does know. Mammogram every year. African America women have stress issues. society does a poor job on stereotypes about African American women
9	13:41.5 - 14:38.8	What are the resources available in your community for breast cancer screening?	Women's clinic. Mammogram center. Mammogram screening. Mobile mammogram machines. Adequate resources.
10	14:38.8 - 15:31.7	Do you how to get available breast cancer screenings?	Receive a letter reminding about 30-60days she is supposed to do mammogram

The top of the page continues the previous row:

cancer screening? (If so, in what ways) — the doctor. They think that their diet is healthy and cannot get it. I can do certain foods I can do abs, I will be fine

		Please describe the process.	
11	15:31.7 - 16:31.2	Have you ever had breast cancer screening? Please explain what type of screening you had and your experience.	She has had screening mammogram. Lifting breasts. at first it was a little sore but machines have become better
12	16:31.2 - 17:46.2	What was the most challenging aspect of breast cancer screening?	First hesitant about showing breasts as it was not modesty. Concern about being bare.
13	17:46.2 - 18:47.5	What factors in your opinion would better enhance your experience and/or utilization of breast cancer screening?	Have another African American woman do it other than a European American female. Because another African American female might understand what you are going though.
14	18:47.5 - 19:19.7	Are you employed and how would you describe your socio-economic status?	Employed. social economic would be considered upper middle class

15	19:19.7 - 19:57.6	Does your socio-economic status influence your breast cancer screening habits?	If you had the money and the insurance resources having more money have influenced her habits
16	19:57.6 - 21:34.6	Do you have health insurance? If no why and if yes, what does your insurance cover?	Has health insurance. United health care. Covers all her medical needs. All inclusive health insurance.
17	21:34.6 - 23:20.4	How affordable is your health insurance, and what factor or factors determined your choice of insurance? How adequate do you think your health insurance is when compared to your health needs	Afford ability of health insurance. Where she works. premiums are very reasonable, very affordable, very adequate health insurance cover
18	23:20.4 - 23:56.5	What is your advice for African American women	Have adequate screening with a health provider

| | | about breast cancer screening? | |

| 19 | 23:56.5 - 24:51.2 | What advice do you have for healthcare providers to improve breast cancer screening services for African American women? | Figure out somewhat to make it accessible and comfortable to go there and no one looks down on them |

| 20 | 24:51.2 - 27:11.0 | Other Comments | Get dialogue from women. Social economic influences. job differences |

Participant 6

	Time span	**Content**	
		Question	**Answer**
1	0:00.0 - 2:26.4	How would you describe your family of origin?	family comes from Liberia but US citizen and has lived in Us for over 40 years
2	2:26.4 - 6:35.2	What do you understand by breast cancer	Prevention is things that you do to stop you from getting breast cancer like screening. Education puts one in a position to do what you need

		prevention and screening?	to do not to get it. Culture to take precaution, voodoo-practicing black medicine. Self education. People don't know the information is available. Able to go to any health care provider and get screening, knows mammogram and self-breast cancer exam. most times the lump is found by oneself
3	6:35.2 - 7:35.9	What concerns do you have about locating and participating in breast cancer screening?	The education is not where it is supposed to do. People do not have an idea and know where they can go to screening. Education is important.
4	7:35.9 - 8:38.4	How does your awareness level about breast cancer screening influence your utilization of the available screening resources?	Always aware that she has to take the initiative to do what she got to do like self examination and education and there are opportunities to participate
5	8:38.4 - 10:31.1	What are your personal barriers that have influenced your breast cancer	Finances, inadequate health insurance because of the present medical condition.

6	10:31.1 - 12:34.0	Do you see culture and stereotype as barriers to breast cancer screening? (If so, in what ways)	Culture that every time somebody dies is due to somebody and nobody dies of natural causes. blacks are more prone to having breast cancer than European American but it is because the European American have access and know better and better health insurance
7	12:34.0 - 13:22.5	What is your attitude and beliefs towards breast cancer screening?	You have to it, you have to initiate it. take every opportunity that you have instead of waiting for the annual screening which you might not go to
8	13:22.5 - 14:37.9	How knowledgeable are you about breast cancer screening recommendations? Please explain	Knowledge from experience and people, who have had breast cancer, has a friend who is going through chemotherapy. they give education and insights and she reads a lot of it
9	14:37.9 - 15:42.4	What are the resources available in your community for	The library, public health facilities, all health care providers have information, TV, Radio, Face book

		breast cancer screening?	
10	15:42.4 - 16:38.6	Do you how to get available breast cancer screenings? Please describe the process.	Starts from gynecologist and her. What she is doing to educate and diet. exposure to sun not necessarily to breast but cancer
11	16:38.6 - 18:31.2	Have you ever had breast cancer screening? Please explain what type of screening you had and your experience.	She has had screening in the sense she had full coverage. Mammogram and everything was okay. but because she does not have insurance and therefore she doesn't do what she would like to do
12	18:31.2 - 19:55.7	What was the most challenging aspect of breast cancer screening?	Mammogram, there could be a more humane way of doing it. It's very traumatic. the process of mammogram
13	19:55.7 - 21:29.6	What factors in your opinion would better enhance your experience and/or utilization of breast cancer screening?	Insurance issues should be taken care of. The method of mammogram is very cruel. it's very painful

14	21:29.6 - 22:58.6	Are you employed and how would you describe your socio-economic status?	Self employed. Work limited due to personal inabilities physical do the work. Financially below the poverty level, which affects her life? But the situation is temporary. hopefully she can go back once it is sorted out
15	22:58.6 - 23:52.0	Does your socio-economic status influence your breast cancer screening habits?	it is affects about mammogram but she does self examination
16	23:52.0 - 24:48.3	Do you have health insurance? If no why and if yes, what does your insurance cover?	I have the affordable care health insurance and she is sure issues have been resolved but she had issues because she had registered twice.
17	24:48.3 - 25:26.6	How affordable is your health insurance, and what factor or factors determined your choice of insurance?	She does not have a choice and she uses what is available to her right now. $150 per month

18	25:26.6 - 26:14.1	How adequate do you think your health insurance is when compared to your health needs	adequate, but right now there is a question whether it should continue, which can get all her health needs met
19	26:14.1 - 27:11.3	What is your advice for African American women about breast cancer screening?	Take energy we have to take care of their health. they should be control of their own health
20	27:11.3 - 28:57.3	What advice do you have for healthcare providers to improve breast cancer screening services for African American women?	You don't have to wait for a gynecologist to do breast screening. All doctors should be equipped to screen. Encourage women to do screening. they should do holistic care
21	28:57.3 - 31:15.4	Other Comments	Initiate own screening and see the doctor, exam should be in reasonable time so that people do not forget. Good to have good health insurance. A little health insurance is better than none. Do follow up and preventive care. Make use of

the resources that they have.

Participant 7

	Time span	Content Question	Answer
1	0:00.0 - 2:10.8	How would you describe your family of origin?	African American, some Indian some Caucasian
2	2:10.8 - 3:19.3	What do you understand by breast cancer prevention and screening?	Screening is very important because early detection is very important. Having a mammogram. self tests by palpating the breasts feeling for lumps
3	3:19.3 - 5:15.7	What concerns do you have about locating and participating in breast cancer screening?	Horror stories she has heard about mammogram. She has had no mammogram. She does self examination. Burning sensation, a radiating pain going across chest, nipples sores and burning a little bit. Within next week or two will go for mammogram, breasts are large and sensitive fearing because of the pain.
4	5:15.7 -	How does your	I know it is available and

	6:57.3	awareness level about breast cancer screening influence your utilization of the available screening resources?	very popular. She has always about it, very aware about what point of life one should be pro active. She is aware of her being over 40 and African American women. aware about where she is supposed to go but she is just making excuses
5	6:57.3 - 10:11.5	What are your personal barriers that have influenced your breast cancer screening behavior?	About being scared about the whole thing. The pain very uncomfortable. The breasts are very large if the breasts weren't so large she would have gone there. But she is going very soon with breasts so large they are flattened like a pancake and has delayed going for screening. fear of unknown
6	10:11.5 - 12:51.5	Do you see culture and stereotype as barriers to breast cancer screening? (If so, in what ways)	Culture and stereotype: social economic status would be a barrier. Low don't go to doctors often. They have low education level. They don't feel that it is self important. They feel that nobody is taking time to educate them. they feel they may dangerous or not comfortable going in there

#	Time	Question	Response
			because of low exposure to education and importance of prevention
7	12:51.5 - 13:44.9	What is your attitude and beliefs towards breast cancer screening?	It is great; the mom had breast cancer and found out. it is well need and screening are available;
8	13:44.9 - 14:52.4	How knowledgeable are you about breast cancer screening recommendations? Please explain	She knows 40 years old mammogram. she didn't go because of fears
9	14:52.4 - 16:39.1	What are the resources available in your community for breast cancer screening? Do you how to get available breast cancer screenings? Please describe the process.	There are doctors. It is not a complicated process. she knows how to get available screening resources
10	16:39.1 - 18:03.2	Have you ever had breast cancer screening? Please	She has had no screening; she is now on the process.

			actually going and seeing what it is about
		explain what type of screening you had and your experience.	
11	18:03.2 - 19:03.1	What was the most challenging aspect of breast cancer screening?	actually going and seeing what it is about
12	19:03.1 - 19:31.4	What factors in your opinion would better enhance your experience and/or utilization of breast cancer screening?	
13	19:31.4 - 21:45.6	Are you employed and how would you describe your socio-economic status?	Self employed. middle class
14	21:45.6 - 22:32.5	Does your socio-economic status influence your breast cancer screening habits?	It should influence, she is well aware but didn't still go. but it could affect someone
15	22:32.5 -	Do you have health insurance? If no why	She doesn't have any insurance because she is

	24:38.5	and if yes, what does your insurance cover? How affordable is your health insurance, and what factor or factors determined your choice of insurance? What is your advice for African American women about breast cancer screening? How adequate do you think your health insurance is when compared to your health needs	self-employed and it is hard but she is streamlining the situation.
16	24:38.5 - 26:21.0	What is your advice for African American women about breast cancer screening?	Advice for African American women. Don't be discouraged, get more information about screening.
17	26:21.0 - 28:03.5	What advice do you have for healthcare providers to improve breast cancer screening services for	Health care providers. Go into the communities educating them. having seminars and go to places where they may not have information

African American
women?

Participant 8

	Time span	Content Question	Answer
1	0:00.0 - 2:00.0	How would you describe your family of origin?	Parents originally from Africa. has lived in Us for more than 40 years
2	2:00.0 - 3:28.7	What do you understand by breast cancer prevention and screening?	At a certain age you have to have your mammogram done and prior to that at age of 20 self examining yourself. Starts at an early age. Look at family history. screening means self examination, mammograms, read literature for other tools
3	3:28.7 - 4:38.8	What concerns do you have about locating and participating in breast cancer screening?	There are available venues to locate to find screening; it's just a matter of looking what is available in your community. No concerns.
4	4:38.8 - 5:38.8	How does your awareness level about breast cancer	. Been around health care for a long time. Because of that knowledge she has

		screening influence your utilization of the available screening resources?	been very aware of that.
5	5:38.8 - 7:15.8	What are your personal barriers that have influenced your breast cancer screening behavior?	Awareness has made it that herself and people around her have screening. You feel that you are a healthy person, eat well, and have no other disease. no family history of breast cancer
6	7:15.8 - 9:00.7	Do you see culture and stereotype as barriers to breast cancer screening? (If so, in what ways)	Not discussed as people think that if you talk about it you get the disease. low-income person and not educated you looked upon at
7	9:00.7 - 9:46.4	What is your attitude and beliefs towards breast cancer screening?	Strongly belief in screening and educating because it can save life
8	9:46.4 - 10:51.1	How knowledgeable are you about breast cancer screening recommendations? Please explain	Knowledgeable about recommendations

9	10:51.1 - 11:53.6	What are the resources available in your community for breast cancer screening?	Clinic in the neighborhood with a breast specialist
10	11:53.6 - 13:16.4	Do you how to get available breast cancer screenings? Please describe the process.	Yes, there are flyers and own physician usually recommends screening.
11	13:16.4 - 14:16.2	Have you ever had breast cancer screening? Please explain what type of screening you had and your experience.	She has had screening. Mammogram yearly. Not the best experience, but the last has been better because the nurses have improved because of more information. it is very painful
12	14:16.2 - 14:50.6	What was the most challenging aspect of breast cancer screening?	Getting the time to schedule it, and mind is how painful the mammogram is
13	14:50.6 - 16:37.7	What factors in your opinion would better enhance your experience and/or	Enhance experience: sensitivity of the technicians doing the screening, understanding

		utilization of breast cancer screening?	how it is painful. Large breasts are painful. Well trained technicians to understand how very painful and difficult it is
14	16:37.7 - 16:59.1	Are you employed and how would you describe your socio-economic status?	employed considered middle class
15	16:59.1 - 17:19.6	Does your socio-economic status influence your breast cancer screening habits?	influences since she has money and insurance she does it
16	17:19.6 - 18:00.3	Do you have health insurance? If no why and if yes, what does your insurance cover?	She has health insurance. it covers some screening but she pays some from her pocket
17	18:00.3 - 18:35.6		Deductible health insurance. Edna Insurance
18	18:35.6 - 19:12.5	How affordable is your health insurance, and what factor or factors determined	payment is very hard, determined by the family member with limited potential

		your choice of insurance?	
19	19:12.5 - 19:46.4	How adequate do you think your health insurance is when compared to your health needs	health insurance covers health needs apart from all screening
20	19:46.4 - 21:15.1	What is your advice for African American women about breast cancer screening?	Be more aware and follow the recommendations of the physicians and have insurance although it's an issue of economics. make it a priority to go for screening
21	21:15.1 - 22:09.7	What advice do you have for healthcare providers to improve breast cancer screening services for African American women?	Offer free screening, team up with insurance companies to screen. making sure the technicians are trained well to reduce pain

Participant 9

Time span	Content Question		Answer

1	0:00.0 - 1:36.0	How would you describe your family of origin?	Immigrant from Nigeria. Lived in America for almost 29years
2	1:38.1 - 2:39.0	What do you understand by breast cancer prevention and screening?	With early detection you can be cured. As a woman you should check every month after monthly periods for self examination, pap smear. do mammogram every year
3	2:39.0 - 5:43.3	What concerns do you have about locating and participating in breast cancer screening?	No concerns have a friend who had been diagnosed ten years now she is okay.
4	5:43.3 - 6:26.2	How does your awareness level about breast cancer screening influence your utilization of the available screening resources?	very knowledgeable . Encourage people and she goes for hers too.
5	6:26.2 - 7:05.6	What are your personal barriers that have influenced your breast cancer screening behavior?	Wish the machine to be warm its cold and she hates the coldness of the mammogram machine

#	Timestamp	Question	Response
6	7:05.6 - 8:58.5	Do you see culture and stereotype as barriers to breast cancer screening? (If so, in what ways)	Culture/stereotype: people are not educated enough, availability of insurance. There is free mammogram but people may not know about it. There are many opportunities. financial barrier
7	8:58.5 - 10:44.5	What is your attitude and beliefs towards breast cancer screening?	apron breast cancer screening
8	10:44.5 - 12:08.7	How knowledgeable are you about breast cancer screening recommendations? Please explain	very knowledgeable
9	12:08.7 - 13:20.4	What are the resources available in your community for breast cancer screening?	Many community activities, free breast screening. Annual Asian festival where there the mammograms. Mobile mammograms. want people to pre register
10	13:20.4 - 16:35.2	Do you how to get available breast cancer	Knows how to get the available resources. Every year using Ohio health mammogram. you can

		screenings? Please describe the process.	walk in and have your mammogram done, she has had mammogram
		Have you ever had breast cancer screening? Please explain what type of screening you had and your experience.	
11	16:35.2 - 19:08.6	What was the most challenging aspect of breast cancer screening?	People complain about breasts being pressed and the coldness of the machine. The experience very nice. don't use perfume or deodorant
		What factors in your opinion would better enhance your experience and/or utilization of breast cancer screening?	
12	19:08.6 - 19:39.6	Are you employed and how would you describe your socio-economic status?	Employed, consider herself comfortable. class between middle class and rich

13	19:39.6 - 20:15.6	Does your socio-economic status influence your breast cancer screening habits?	social economic status influences because she is knowledgeable and have medical insurance coverage
14	20:15.6 - 21:40.6	Do you have health insurance? If no why and if yes, what does your insurance cover?	Has health care insurance. Covers mammogram fully, utilize mammogram. optimal health insurance, part of Ohio health
15	21:40.6 - 23:37.4	How affordable is your health insurance, and what factor or factors determined your choice of insurance? How adequate do you think your health insurance is when compared to your health needs	Affordable, does not have a choice but she would go with the lowest pay. look at afford ability, very adequate health insurance
16	23:37.4 - 27:54.1	What is your advice for African American women about breast cancer screening?	People should screen no matter the family history and age. Do self examination usually after the period or date of your birthday if you are

			menopausal. go for screening even after mastectomy
17	27:54.1 - 29:45.8	What advice do you have for healthcare providers to improve breast cancer screening services for African American women?	Education, promote primary prevention
18	29:45.8 - 32:04.3	Other Comments	have posters that show how to do self-examination to be hang in the bathroom

Participant 10

	Time span	Content Question	Answer
1	0:00.0 - 1:26.1	How would you describe your family of origin?	mother and father African born in Africa and became us citizen been America for more than 40 years
2	1:26.1 - 2:28.6	What do you understand by breast cancer prevention and screening?	Doing what you need to do to prevent through mammogram and self examination. Having a regular doctor to direct you to mammogram, self-breast

			examination is recommended. doesn't do it regularly
3	2:28.6 - 4:03.3	What concerns do you have about locating and participating in breast cancer screening?	Every woman there is one of those things you don't want to find. Fearful concern. don't have any problem finding screening services
4	4:03.3 - 5:52.7	How does your awareness level about breast cancer screening influence your utilization of the available screening resources?	Very privileged by working in oncology nursing. involved in teaching and educating women and because of that it has increased awareness, very aware of location and need which encourages her to continue
5	5:52.7 - 6:45.8	What are your personal barriers that have influenced your breast cancer screening behavior?	laziness and forgetfulness, and making time
6	6:45.8 - 10:10.8	Do you see culture and stereotype as barriers to breast	Probably not. Some of friends and people she interacts with think it's not important, some of them do not have health care

		cancer screening? (If so, in what ways)	insurance, African not taught to do it culturally. Stereotype is hard for her to say. It is based on individual need. how do her as a woman is good for her
7	10:10.8 - 11:31.0	What is your attitude and beliefs towards breast cancer screening?	Screening is important. Do concern themselves get exposed to. is it important to do mammogram every year
8	11:31.0 - 12:53.9	How knowledgeable are you about breast cancer screening recommendations? Please explain	she knows about the recommendation of doing it every single year
9	12:53.9 - 13:46.2	What are the resources available in your community for breast cancer screening?	Knowledge and awareness of the resources available through the doctor through the community. There are free services for breast cancer exam.
10	13:46.2 - 15:13.0	Do you how to get available breast cancer screenings? Please describe the process.	If you have a doctor he should recommend. if you have a doctor or insurance you can go to a free clinic and ask for free mammogram screening

#	Time	Question	Response
11	15:13.0 - 16:03.1	Have you ever had breast cancer screening? Please explain what type of screening you had and your experience.	Self examination and mammogram. two or three of them they found something which was scary but found it was some tissues
12	16:03.1 - 17:32.5	What was the most challenging aspect of breast cancer screening?	Waiting when they said they found something was scary was very scary. The experience called booby smashing, the cold. it doesn't bother her but wishes it was warmer
13	17:32.5 - 18:06.2	What factors in your opinion would better enhance your experience and/or utilization of breast cancer screening?	warm equipment and nice personality,
14	18:06.2 - 18:22.4	Are you employed and how would you describe your socio-economic status?	employed, comfortable, not rich not poor
15	18:22.4 - 19:21.4	Does your socio-economic status	Its hard question, she doesn't know what she could do if

		influence your breast cancer screening habits?	she did not have the resources. economic does not affect the decision
16	19:21.4 - 20:05.7	Do you have health insurance? If no why and if yes, what does your insurance cover?	she has health insurance and coverage is okay
17	20:05.7 - 20:40.9	How affordable is your health insurance, and what factor or factors determined your choice of insurance?	Did not have choice for the type of insurance. it is expensive but they have to pay
18	20:40.9 - 21:00.6	How adequate do you think your health insurance is when compared to your health needs	very adequate health insurance
19	21:00.6 - 23:37.9	What is your advice for African American women about breast cancer screening?	No matter how people view you, you got have to look at you and decide you need to take care of yourself health wise. There are resources there and they need to tap into the resources available.

			If you value who you are you have to make the decision to do what you can to save you. ask each other whether they have done their mammogram
20	23:37.9 - 24:47.6	What advice do you have for healthcare providers to improve breast cancer screening services for African American women?	When you see a woman in the clinic. have the initial assessment to ask when did you do your last mammogram exam as admission assessment
21	24:47.6 - 26:23.1	Other Comments	teach new nurses to know how to do good assessment to do from head to toe

Participant 11

	Time span	Content Question	Answer
1	0:00.0 - 1:57.7	How would you describe your family of origin?	Black American. Parents from Africa. she has been America for many years
2	1:57.7 - 2:55.0	What do you understand by breast	A way of checking the breasts either by oneself or through mammogram.

		cancer prevention and screening?	she knows self examination looking for lumps in the breasts
3	2:55.0 - 3:49.1	What concerns do you have about locating and participating in breast cancer screening?	It is very necessary but most of them are limited because of the cost as majority of women have no insurance to cover mammogram
4	3:49.1 - 5:56.5	How does your awareness level about breast cancer screening influence your utilization of the available screening resources?	She is aware of the screening it's good and its need but because she doesn't have insurance to cover herself she does self assessment. and belief that God will take control especially when there is no finance
5	5:56.5 - 6:59.6	What are your personal barriers that have influenced your breast cancer screening behavior?	Time, no insurance to cover the bill. now that she knows there could be free testing she will find a place
6	6:59.6 - 9:18.9	Do you see culture and stereotype as barriers to breast cancer screening? (If so, in what ways)	Culture is a barrier because most African American women she is grandmother and helps look after the granddaughter so she

#	Time	Question	Response
			doesn't have time. Beliefs that God will be in control. African Americans do care it's because of time and finances are the barriers
7	9:18.9 - 10:03.6	What is your attitude and beliefs towards breast cancer screening?	Very important to go for screening, that is mammogram for early detection.
8	10:03.6 - 11:04.3	How knowledgeable are you about breast cancer screening recommendations? Please explain	She knows that she should check herself after bathing even there are any lumps. does not know about mammogram and that there are free mammograms
9	11:04.3 - 12:52.5	What are the resources available in your community for breast cancer screening?	She does not really know about the resources available. Daughter told her about mammogram, and she does not want anybody to see or touch her breasts and did not know about the seriousness.

10	12:52.5 - 13:17.4	Do you how to get available breast cancer screenings? Please describe the process.	she does not know how to find available resources
11	13:17.4 - 14:19.6	Have you ever had breast cancer screening? Please explain what type of screening you had and your experience.	She does self-examination but has not gone through mammogram. she stands in front of the mirror and checks for lumps
12	14:19.6 - 15:13.1	What was the most challenging aspect of breast cancer screening?	she does not have any challenges in self-examination but does not remember to do it most times
13	15:13.1 - 16:12.5	What factors in your opinion would better enhance your experience and/or utilization of breast cancer screening?	Free tests could enhance her participation for people to just walk in and advertise it the way they do it about smoking and gun. more awareness
14	16:12.5 - 16:59.6	Are you employed and how would you describe your socio-economic status?	Employed part time but her social status, she is being helped by her daughter as well therefore

			comfortable.
15	16:59.6 - 17:19.2	Does your socio-economic status influence your breast cancer screening habits?	social economic status affects because she does not have insurance and keeps away from mammogram because she cannot afford it
16	17:19.2 - 17:50.1	Do you have health insurance? If no why and if yes, what does your insurance cover?	Doesn't have health insurance. By December she will have health insurance from the place she works.
		How affordable is your health insurance, and what factor or factors determined your choice of insurance?	
		How adequate do you think your health insurance is when compared to your health needs	
17	17:50.1 - 18:49.8	What is your advice for African American	African American women should come out in masses and go for mammogram because it is very

	Time span	Content Question	Answer
		women about breast cancer screening?	important. No what is happening and take care of themselves. stop believing that God will do it but do what you have to do
18	18:51.4 - 22:15.0	What advice do you have for healthcare providers to improve breast cancer screening services for African American women?	They should make available the mammogram screening free because people don't participate because they cannot afford it. go to the rural areas where there are more grandmother and grandfathers and provide awareness and provide free screening
19	22:15.0 - 24:07.0	Other Comments	She did not agree with her daughter when she was told about screening but now, she believes and will let other people know about it.

Participant 12

Time span	Content Question	Answer

1	0:00.0 - 1:30.6	How would you describe your family of origin?	Fore father came from Nigeria. but African American
2	1:30.6 - 2:40.9	What do you understand by breast cancer prevention and screening?	The area you screen is better to prevent, exercise, eating well. Helps well to prevent breast cancer. Most important is screening for early detection. self-examination and doing mammogram every year
3	2:40.9 - 5:02.3	What concerns do you have about locating and participating in breast cancer screening?	The only place that she knows of is going to the hospital and the center. More locations like in the supermarkets, schools. no problem locating the screening resources
4	5:02.3 - 6:10.1	How does your awareness level about breast cancer screening influence your utilization of the available screening resources?	being a nurse, she knows that the screening is very important and does not miss any yearly mammogram screening
5	6:10.1 - 7:58.9	What are your personal barriers that	Every time after finishing screening, the way they mash the breasts, pressing

		have influenced your breast cancer screening behavior?	it is painful. How they manipulate the breasts turning it here and there, lifting it up. it invades your privacy
6	7:58.9 - 9:33.2	Do you see culture and stereotype as barriers to breast cancer screening? (If so, in what ways)	Africans don't belief in health care much. They believe they are okay. Too busy to go and check themselves up. As long as they are well, they think that they do not need it. no education, no money or insurance
7	9:33.2 - 10:37.8	What is your attitude and beliefs towards breast cancer screening?	The screening is very important. encourages her girls to do self-assessment and she encourages people of her age to go for screening
8	10:37.8 - 11:34.2	How knowledgeable are you about breast cancer screening recommendations? Please explain	Self-examination every month. 40 years and above should go to screening. if you notice anything strange go to the doctor
9	11:34.2 - 12:09.4	What are the resources available in	Mobile screening centers but not often. would be nice to get more of that

		your community for breast cancer screening?	
10	12:09.4 - 13:09.7	Do you how to get available breast cancer screenings? Please describe the process.	She knows how to get available screening resources. When she goes for pap smear, he always sends her for mammogram. screening through her doctor (OBGY)
11	13:09.7 - 15:03.4	Have you ever had breast cancer screening? Please explain what type of screening you had and your experience.	She has had self-examination and mammogram. The pressing is so hard, touching and playing with your breasts. it's okay but she would prefer somebody not touching or playing with her breasts
12	15:03.4 - 15:50.5	What was the most challenging aspect of breast cancer screening?	Touching, pulling, and smashing that you are uncomfortable for some times. the temperatures are cold the nipples are pointing
13	15:50.5 - 17:06.1	What factors in your opinion would better enhance your	Participants play with their own breasts and not other people doing it. The

		experience and/or utilization of breast cancer screening?	temperatures should not be very cold. although she would still go for it
14	17:06.1 - 18:18.7	Are you employed and how would you describe your socio-economic status?	She is employed with full time job. she in the middle-class status and married, stable not rich nor poor
15	18:18.7 - 19:15.9	Does your socio-economic status influence your breast cancer screening habits?	the social economic status helps since she has insurance that pay part of it
16	19:15.9 - 19:38.7	Do you have health insurance? If no why and if yes, what does your insurance cover?	the insurance covers about 80% and she pays 20%
17	19:38.7 - 20:35.3		United Health care. A co pay that when she visits about$15, dental, vision, health care. co pay is not bad at all
18	20:35.3 - 21:37.6	How affordable is your health insurance, and what factor or factors determined	the insurance is through a husband from the place he works and well affordable

	Time span	Question	Answer
		your choice of insurance?	
19	21:37.6 - 22:39.2	How adequate do you think your health insurance is when compared to your health needs	insurance is adequate for their health needs, she is happy with the insurance
20	22:39.2 - 23:47.9	What is your advice for African American women about breast cancer screening?	African American women should make the screening possible even if it means scheduling it around their birthdays. education is more important
21	23:47.9 - 26:26.0	What advice do you have for healthcare providers to improve breast cancer screening services for African American women?	Having mammogram day for free for anybody to come in and participate. more education about examination and screening

Participant 13

Time span	Contents Question	Answer

1	0:00.0 - 1:29.5	How would you describe your family of origin?	African American. mum and dad blacks from US
2	1:29.5 - 2:02.6	What do you understand by breast cancer prevention and screening?	every woman 45 years old and older should have mammogram per year and self-examination regularly
3	2:02.6 - 2:08.9	What concerns do you have about locating and participating in breast cancer screening?	no concerns
4	2:08.9 - 3:13.1	How does your awareness level about breast cancer screening influence your utilization of the available screening resources?	Being a nurse she is very aware of the importance of screening. It's very important for her to go yearly and she has gone to the same clinic, and she is much supported.
5	3:13.1 - 3:51.4	What are your personal barriers that have influenced your breast cancer screening behavior?	No barriers. her mum was very health conscious, and she was pushing them to have information
6	3:51.4 - 4:28.2	Do you see culture and stereotype as barriers to	Black women do not think that breast cancer affects them. Younger

#	Time	Question	Response
		breast cancer screening? (If so, in what ways)	inner-city women don't think about it. there is stereotype that only European American women get it
7	4:28.2 - 5:48.6	What is your attitude and beliefs towards breast cancer screening?	It is something that all women should be very cognitive off. all the years when she did not think about breast cancer with early detection, they have a better chance of survival
8	5:48.6 - 6:35.3	How knowledgeable are you about breast cancer screening recommendations? Please explain	Very knowledgeable about recommendations. It's everywhere. There is a month for breast screening. they need to open up their eyes and see
9	6:35.3 - 7:05.2	What are the resources available in your community for breast cancer screening?	Women's health clinic. mobile clinic
10	7:05.2 - 8:13.2	Do you how to get available breast cancer	she knows the process to get available screening resources, she has done self-examination since

		screenings? Please describe the process.	she was in her early 20s
11	8:13.2 - 8:33.3	Have you ever had breast cancer screening? Please explain what type of screening you had and your experience.	first mammogram was very painful
12	8:33.3 - 8:58.8	What was the most challenging aspect of breast cancer screening?	Having her breasts squeezed in that machine. she did not like it at all
13	8:58.8 - 9:35.9	What factors in your opinion would better enhance your experience and/or utilization of breast cancer screening?	Being explained to how it is done before actually going for screening about experience. make machine not hurt
14	9:35.9 - 9:44.7	Are you employed and how would you describe your socio-economic status?	Employed. middle class
15	9:44.7 - 10:15.7	Does your socio-economic status influence your breast cancer screening habits?	Doesn't affect it. she is educated because she had a mum who was very aware

16	10:15.7 - 10:31.7	Do you have health insurance? If no why and if yes, what does your insurance cover?	health insurance covers wellness visits
17	10:31.7 - 11:03.3		United health care covers almost everything. 20% co pay
18	11:03.3 - 11:55.6	How affordable is your health insurance, and what factor or factors determined your choice of insurance?	Cost is not too horrible for her. Factors determining is what it covers. the job dictates the insurance
19	11:55.6 - 12:17.6	How adequate do you think your health insurance is when compared to your health needs	very adequate
20	12:17.6 - 13:16.0	What is your advice for African American women about breast cancer screening?	have screening done because early detection there is a chance for survival
21	13:16.0 - 14:41.6	What advice do you have for healthcare providers	Always have provision for screening even if one does not have that

		to improve breast cancer screening services for African American women?	expensive insurance. provide for all women despite the insurance they carry
22	14:41.6 - 15:38.0	Other Comments	have conversations and encourage them to have screening and educate them

Participant 14

	Time span	Content Question	Answer
1	0:00.0 - 1:31.9	How would you describe your family of origin?	From Africa. Parents born from the western part of Africa. she has lived in America for many years
2	1:31.9 - 2:37.2	What do you understand by breast cancer prevention and screening?	breast cancer is a rampant disease screening is part of preventive methods and has many benefits like discovering it early and the cancer of curing it is more possible than developed stage
3	2:37.2 - 3:18.2	What concerns do you have about locating and participating in	Don't have any concerns she knows where to go. she knows there are people limited by many

		breast cancer screening?	reasons like lack of insurance, lack of proximity, lack of knowledge as to where to go
4	3:18.2 - 4:23.8	How does your awareness level about breast cancer screening influence your utilization of the available screening resources?	She believes she is very aware and that is what influences her utilization. she pays attention to the time she did it and the time to do it again and find a place ahead of time for screening
5	4:23.8 - 4:54.8	What are your personal barriers that have influenced your breast cancer screening behavior?	no personal barriers she believes that she gets advantage of opportunities available
6	4:54.8 - 6:00.4	Do you see culture and stereotype as barriers to breast cancer screening? (If so, in what ways)	Sometimes people think themselves as belonging to a family with no history of cancer and assuming that it cannot happen and thus ignore opportunities. they think they don't need it
7	6:00.4 - 6:44.4	What is your attitude and beliefs towards	A very important thing to do. Doesn't matter what your experience has been

		breast cancer screening?	even if no other person in your family. its go to go and find out nothing than not going and there is something
8	6:44.4 - 8:04.9	How knowledgeable are you about breast cancer screening recommendations? Please explain	Knowledgeable enough she knows that women should do self-examination and do yearly mammograms
9	8:04.9 - 8:52.7	What are the resources available in your community for breast cancer screening?	aware that there are clinics, can get information from family doctors, specialist doctors, insurance covers screening, mobile units
10	8:52.7 - 9:08.1		
11	9:08.1 - 9:47.5	Do you how to get available breast cancer screenings? Please describe the process.	She knows how that one should call the providers and schedule an appointment and bring things you asked to and be there in time.
12	9:47.5 - 10:45.0	Have you ever had breast cancer screening? Please	Several mammograms in the few years. Have had pleasant experience. has utilized mobile unit

		explain what type of screening you had and your experience.	
13	10:45.0 - 11:14.9	What was the most challenging aspect of breast cancer screening?	Getting started was the most challenging thing.
14	11:12.2 - 12:02.1	What factors in your opinion would better enhance your experience and/or utilization of breast cancer screening?	It's good as it is. the pressing of breasts sometimes is work
15	12:02.1 - 12:28.5	Are you employed and how would you describe your socio-economic status?	employed and middle class
16	12:28.5 - 13:15.3	Does your socio-economic status influence your breast cancer screening habits?	The status has made her realize importance. people she associates with believe that it is important
17	13:15.3 - 13:39.4	Do you have health insurance? If no why	she has health insurance that covers virtually

		and if yes, what does your insurance cover?	everything
18	13:39.4 - 13:57.0		cooperative health insurance provided through her job and united health care
19	13:57.0 - 14:41.4	How affordable is your health insurance, and what factor or factors determined your choice of insurance?	determined by her job, the insurance is affordable because the employer pays the bunch
20	14:41.4 - 15:33.9	How adequate do you think your health insurance is when compared to your health needs	Very adequate. she pays a co pay
21	15:33.9 - 17:51.1	What is your advice for African American women about breast cancer screening?	Screening is necessary for every woman especially after the age of 40. There is a tendency of thinking that it is hereditary and hence they do not go for screening because they think they are safe, do screening regularly. Don't do self-examination as frequently as required.

| 22 | 17:51.1 -
19:29.1 | What advice do you have for healthcare providers to improve breast cancer screening services for African American women? | take it seriously

Make the atmosphere friendly. Creating services that will bring screening closer to the communities might be a useful thing to do. finding government funding so as the services can be made free |

www.ingramcontent.com/pod-product-compliance
Lightning Source LLC
Chambersburg PA
CBHW051514150726
47997CB00001B/248